TIME OUT OF MIND

TIME OUT OF MIND

Jane Lapotaire

CHIVERS

British Library Cataloguing in Publication Data available

This Large Print edition is published by BBC Audiobooks Ltd, England,

Published in 2004 in the U.K. by arrangement with Time Warner Books Ltd

U.K. Hardcover ISBN 0-7540-9902 4
U.K. Softcover   ISBN 0-7540-9903 2

The text of this Large Print edition is unabridged.
Other aspects of the book may vary from the original edition.

Set in 16 pt. New Times Roman.

Printed in Great Britain on acid-free paper.

362
196
811

La

For Ger

Printed and bound in Great Britain by
Antony Rowe Ltd., Chippenham, Wiltshire

Acknowledgements

Special thanks to: Dr Vinikoff and the neuro-surgical team at the Hôpital Lariboisière, Paris, who saved my life; Mr Neil Kitchen, who read the manuscript; Dr Eliane Miotto of the National Hospital for Neurology and Neurosurgery, London; Dr George Lewith, Homeopath, Acupuncturist; Dr Keith McKee, GP; Renata Symonds, Jungian analyst; the Reverend Dr Martin Israel; Peter Overton, MRO, and Dr Jovan Djurovic, osteopaths; and Judith Seelig, all of whom helped me with their healing skills, and showed me care and understanding during this difficult time. My thanks too for financial support from the Royal Shakespeare Company, the Royal Theatrical Fund and the King George V Fund for Actors and Actresses.

To the few friends whose patience my new brain tested to the utmost and who still stuck by me—they know who they are—my heartfelt gratitude.

To my agents at 'Storm', Sam, Jo and Tig, for believing in my recovery against all odds.

To Lennie Goodings and Elise Dillsworth at Virago without whom this would have been but half a book.

But most of all to those I couldn't have pulled through without: Sandra Buckley and the BASIC helpline; Dr Sherrie Baehr, Neuropsychologist at the Rehabilitation Network, who also read the manuscript; my son, Rowan, for whom this was an enormous ordeal, and to the Godsend, who really gave me a new life— my love.

CONTENTS

When one is a stranger to oneself then one is estranged from others too.

VITA SACKVILLE-WEST

On bad days I wish I had died on that volcano with Igor and the others. Many times my wife has said that the old me did die that day on Galeras. She's right. I am not the same. I was always an impatient and aggressive person, but courtesy and normal inhibitions kept me in check. After the head injury, however, the brakes on my bad behaviour seemed to fail and I found myself barking at my wife and losing my temper over the smallest things. Slowly I pushed her away. As the doctors reconstructed me, I joked that I was like Frankenstein. Now I occasionally look in the mirror and wonder, 'Who is this monster?' My frustrations have been compounded by a powerful mixture of seizure medications and anti-depressants. 'You were put back together like Humpty Dumpty and patted on the back and told your recovery was impressive,' she wrote to me recently. ' "You are so lucky your husband has recovered so well," people tell me. That phrase haunts me as countless people tell me how lucky I am you survived.' I am so tired of people pretending everything is fine when it's not. Only those who have lived with ambivalent loss can understand this . . .

STANLEY WILLAMS, Surviving Galeras

Surgeons must be careful
When they ply the knife
Underneath their fine incisions
Stirs the culprit Life.
                    EMILY DICKINSON

Pain is normally the enemy of the descriptive powers. Daudet discovered that pain (like passion) drives out language. Words come only when everything is over.
                    JULIAN BARNES, *Alphonse Daudet*

AUTHOR'S NOTE

On 11 January 2000 I collapsed with what was eventually diagnosed as a burst middle cerebral artery aneurysm. I spent three and a half largely unconscious weeks in Intensive Care recovering from the six-hour operation to clip the aneurysm, and two angioplasty operations to prevent the brain subsequently going into spasm, which can cause a massive blockage of blood, which means death.

This book is an attempt to explain to myself what happened in the days and months that followed, as time and experience became alien to me. It is also an attempt to describe the journey to recovery in a subjective manner using the skills and techniques of my craft as an actor, to give those who have suffered a similar experience, a voice. (It might perhaps be fitting to describe it as making a drama out of a crisis.)

Unlike recovery from strokes (which is largely visible) once the scar has healed and the hair regrown after a cerebral haemorrhage, the experience, as I continually discover, was at worst totally foreign to most people and at best misunderstood. The brain is left vulnerable to noise, physical jostling or any form of vocal and emotional harshness. This book, I hope, will also be of help to those who watch their loved ones struggle to come to terms with their lives being irretrievably changed after a subarachnoid haemorrhage, and for us, the brain-damaged, the challenge of getting to know a stranger: ourselves.

Introduction

It is New Year's Eve 1999. I arrive at my ex-husband's home, early. This large house in Chelsea, with its imposing pillars at either side of the porch, is where I used to live twenty years ago with him and our son. They are inside now making ready for the evening meal, with his second wife, my son's stepmother of some six years. I don't want the evening to start yet, so I decide to take a walk. That in itself is odd. I can't remember the last time I had a few unrushed moments to myself.

The streets are dark and strangely silent. People are indoors preparing for the evening's celebrations. I peer through many windows where candles flicker and tables are laid with glinting glasses, crisp fancy-folded napkins and shiny plates. Decorations on Christmas trees reflect the dance of the flames in nearby fires. These are the streets where I used to walk our son in his pushchair. I know them well. I sit for a while in the Catholic church where an early service is progressing. I often used to seek refuge in the silent coolness of this church, kept out from the heart of it by the bars that shuttered its gilded ornaments from thieving hands, my baby son on my knee. I am kept out now, although the barred gates are pushed open. I remain distant from the mass. The

1

repetitions sound just that to me. Words repeated without any meaning, any conviction. I can find nothing real behind the gold and the paint. It may be that the theatre gives me all I need from ritual, and that I must search for the Divine beyond image, in something simpler. To put it another way, I've always been a bolshie stubborn sod. Never liked isms. Never belonged to any group or faction. Always wanted to make my own mistakes. I make one concession as I leave quietly. I cross myself. I hope no one sees. I have crossed myself in the Greek Orthodox way, as I do on stage.

I am playing Maria Callas on tour round the provinces of England, hoping that as, apparently, the reviews have been excellent, we will eventually make it into the West End. I love her dearly. There is a heart-stopping moment in every performance as the first aria bleeds through the amplifiers into the dialogue I am speaking. With the piercing clarity of those first notes, I feel her spirit come into the theatre to join me on stage. It is a privilege to play her. Most times I feel she plays me. It is also excruciatingly exhausting. I have to motor two and a quarter hours of play virtually single-handed. I spent four long months researching her life, her character, her career, her clothes, her friends, her habits, before starting the arduous rehearsals. I learned the arias by heart in Italian, the arias she teaches

2

in the play. She only has to sing one line and that badly. This is the one aspect of the play for which I didn't have to do research or have any lessons. She is passionate, clever, a musical genius and a fine actress. The first who really combined the two great disciplines of Acting and Opera. She is, as Piaf was (whom I also played), a *monstre sacré*. Her personal grandeur, and the rigour with which she teaches the two sopranos and the tenor in the play, *Masterclass*, have detached me from the rest of the cast. They are young and largely inexperienced, and find it difficult to know where Callas stops and I begin. So it is an isolated time. We have done eight gruelling weeks, with another eight to go. There is a break over Christmas and the New Year while stages are filled with pantomimes, so I shall go and teach a Shakespeare masterclass. I have taught for over fifteen years in England and America, but this, unusually, as it happens, is in Paris. It will help ease the expense of touring and running a home in London on a non-West End salary.

I walk towards the Albert Bridge, my favourite bridge in London. I love its fine white iron tracery, its palest pink circles and yellowy cream whorls. It reminds me of a delicate ornamental wedding cake. I harbour a fancy of living near this bridge. It would be good to be so near my ex-husband's house: my son often stays there. His father and

3

stepmother live most of the year in Los Angeles. This get-together on New Year's Eve has become almost an annual event , although recurrence hasn't made it easier. I go to give my son a chance of seeing his parents together, albeit briefly. He was five when I took him from this house and left.

I stop and look down into the blackness of the river, then up into the star-dotted darkness. There is hardly anyone about yet. It feels odd. Later, I don't doubt, the river will be full of boats and reflections of fireworks, the pavements thick with throngs of people, us among them. I drink in the darkness. A night off during the run of a play always holds a special relish, and that this night is the last of the millennium gives it an added patina. For a few seconds, time stands still. I feel very quiet deep inside. I have every intention of holding on to this rare serenity. I will need it to see me through the evening. I think back over the year just a little, not too much, I don't want to threaten this mood. My mother died in March. Two days after my son's birthday. The mother I never lived with. The French mother who left me in Suffolk at two months old, to be fostered by the old lady who, for twelve of my mother's nineteen years as an orphan from Barnardo's, had fostered her. I was terrified that she would die on the actual day of my son's birthday and, as a consequence, blight that day for me for ever. I was terrified of my mother. And not

4

just during my childhood. Most children who were unwanted are convinced that the fault is theirs. I am no exception. I have spent most of my fifty-five years learning to recognise this deep conviction in all its ever-changing guises. As I look up into the sky I wonder where her spirit is. I suspect, because of her nature and the nature of her life, that wherever it is, it is unlikely to be at rest. I look down into the liquid darkness again: little eddies of empty bottles and rubbish swirl around in the tide. I look where the river imperceptibly meets the dark horizon. I hear one of the lines from the play, which Callas shouts after the retreating Onassis: 'Don't leave me. I've been alone all my life until now.'

Later that evening as my son and his stepmother weave their way back through the crowds just ahead of us, with his beautiful girlfriend and a zany friend of hers who's wielding a bright neon pink wand with a star at its tip, my ex-husband puts his arm round me and says, 'And how are *you*, Janie?'

Swarms of explanations buzz about my brain, all of them inadequate to describe my present state. I am disturbed by his nearness. 'Tired to my bones,' I say. But words can't go that deep.

I leave not long after two o'clock, stone cold sober, and drive back to the little terraced house in Putney where I live alone now that my son has grown up and gone.

For some unaccountable reason, days later in a frenzy of cleaning up, I turn out all the diaries and notebooks I kept during my marriage and my son's early years. Well, I'm going to work in America for nine months later this new year. That's clearing out and making space.

But what I can't explain is why, after not having seen him for twenty years, I visit my solicitor and bring my will up to date.

CHAPTER ONE

Nearly Dying Is the Easy Bit

11 January 2000

I wake feeling ghastly. Nothing new in that. I've woken feeling ghastly for years. Tired, achy, lifeless, all symptoms of overwork. This is and has been the norm for about eight years. The only not-norm is that I've woken feeling ghastly in Paris. A grey wintry Paris. Grey in spite of the wickedly flashing pink lights on the Eiffel Tower, whose top is just visible from a friend of a friend's balcony and who, in the pink ruffles of her skirt below, tells me we are eleven days into the new millennium. It is a date I will remember.

I eat breakfast of wheat-free *biscottes* and black coffee, and wonder with which of the painkillers to punctuate the coffee—which of the cocktail from my bathroom cupboard has found its way into my overnight case. I have painkillers in every piece of luggage I possess. Like most performers I have physical injuries from my job—back problems, neck problems and regular headaches, which of course come from the back and neck problems. I have painkillers with muscle relaxant, painkillers that give me a lift, and painkillers with sleep aid. Today I need pills that mask the ache in my body, fool me into thinking I'm OK, and give me some semblance of energy with which to teach this all-day Shakespeare masterclass for sixteen- and eighteen-year-olds, usually not the most willing of captive audiences, at the École Internationale de Paris, just across the other side of the road and a bit further down the rue de Passy. I gratefully swallow two Aleve from my American arsenal—you can't buy them in England. As I orbit out of the warmth of the little clanking wooden lift, past the swirling thirties staircase into the greyness, I say to Ann, who organises my teaching work and has travelled with me, 'I'll just have my last cigarette.' It was.

Later, I'm thinking as I chew gum, hoping to mask the smell of the smoke, and try to ignore the *chic* of all the passers-by, and their occasional look of disapproval, how my mother would have disapproved of my smoking in the street. This is after all, the 16*ième*. Posh it may be, I concede grudgingly, in reply to her in my head, but in spite of its nearness to the Bois de Boulogne—Callas, who is much on what's left of my mind, lived not far away, and walked her beloved dogs there—this *arrondissement* seems all concrete and grey stone to me. Paris could never be austere, but this area is rather sombre and grand. I'd rather be in the only little bit of Paris I know at all, on the Left Bank. Then I

8

realise this is the first time I have set foot in France since my mother died. It is almost nine months to the day. How odd.

Some half-hour later I'm standing in the middle of the school gym, which is lined with talkative young faces, bright from the cold and, I hope, expectation of our day together. They are probably more excited by the relief that they've escaped their normal classes, and are chattering away in a variety of English and American accents. These are mostly children of diplomat and business parents whose work keeps them in Paris; the school keeps them within the American education system. I'm not quite sure where I fit into that, other than I hope they'll see me as a sort of fun day off. It'd be a bonus if any of them should feel marginally less bored or terrified of Shakespeare. I'm aware of the smell that all school gyms have, and this one is no exception: that distinctive mixture of young bodies, old trainers and trapped sweat. The school's head, a likeable Welsh chap, calls for silence and proceeds to introduce me in a very complimentary manner. I'm planning, when he finishes, on making a joke similar to the one I sometimes make in these circumstances: why doesn't he give up being a headmaster, since he sees my career in such a benevolent light, and become my agent? Today I never get to make the joke.

I stop listening to his voice as I become

9

aware slowly that the world has gone wavy. Nothing is solid. I think I'm going to faint. I think, My God, I am, I'm going to faint. I don't faint. It's not something I do. I have never fainted in my life. Get the water, I think. I move, I hope, towards the glass of water. Waves tip the floor from under my feet, ripple the walls and faces in front of my eyes, undulate along my spine and engulf me. Time goes awry.

I am looking at a large white bowl very near my face, full of bright orange stuff. I retch some more. So that's what gluten-free *biscottes* and black coffee look like, I muse. Months later I wonder if it was the blood from my brain that stained my breakfast vivid orange.

Colours leap out at me. Time becomes black and silent. Viscous. Orange. Grey and silent. Or, much later, bright cobalt blue.

I am filled with love for the tall, dark-haired men from SAMU (Service d'Assistance Medicale d'Urgence) who are busy around me. I never want them to stop whatever they are doing for me. I have no idea where I am or what is going on, and no interest in it either.

I have no memory of talking at all, but I do remember a dry scraping sound above me, intermingled with shadow then brightness. The dry *kkkkk, kkkk, kkkk* comes from a circular disc on the roof that slowly turns and intermittently blots out an orange light. My head is fitted into something that feels like a padded helmet, with such gentleness that again I am overwhelmed. These men are so dark they could be from the Languedoc. Or perhaps they're Basques. I remember the home I had in the Languedoc once. I hear the *pam-pom pam-pom* of the ambulance. The sound seems so near. My whole body jumps and bumps up and down. I am rattled over what must be the cobbles of the streets of Paris. Someone nearby is shouting, 'My head, my head.' I wonder who it is. Blackness.

I open my eyes. All is grey. Calm, neutral grey. I can distinguish nothing. A door opens in the greyness and my son comes in. On automatic maternal pilot I say, 'Don't worry about the train fare. I'll give you the money back for the train fare,' and close my eyes again.

A man with a serene face and deep dark eyes seems to be sitting on my bed. I think I'm still in the ambulance but I'm not. It's now Friday (I find out weeks later) and they're going to operate. I'm at the Hôpital Lariboisière, where the first hospital sent me on the Tuesday I collapsed, after they'd scanned me from head to toe and discovered I was bleeding in my brain. The surgeon, he with the deep dark eyes, explains very slowly and carefully, as if talking to a child, that it is a very serious thing that has happened to me, and that the operation is very serious indeed, and my chances of pulling through are slight. He tells me his name, then asks me if I have understood. I tell him I have. Then he asks me to repeat his name. 'Docteur Vinikoff,' I say, proud that I have got it right. He reminds me of my ex-husband. He smiles at me and I am filled with a rush of benevolence and well-being.

Ann, who has been by my side apparently for the four days since the incident, who coped with my being unconscious, held the bowl for me to be sick in, undressed me, took my hearing-aid out and my rings and necklace off, sits solemnly to my left. 'Do you realise you might die?' she says, or something like that, reminding me that, on her own admission, her French is atrocious. She would have understood little of what Vinikoff had said. There is something more grave about hearing the words in English.

I think, I'm glad I've been an actor. It's given me glimpses of life I would never have had. I hear myself say, 'I've had a good life. I've met some interesting people and been to some extraordinary places.' There seems to be no more to say, though even at the time I think, That sounds so banal. I have no sense of moving towards the Divine or anything like that. I don't even pray. I am pervaded by an overwhelming sense of acceptance, calm and

12

peace. I think, So that's *that* then, and then I say, 'Tell my son I love him.' And not wanting her to feel left out I add, 'And you, Ann, and you.'

Dr Vinikoff seems to be sitting on my bed again. Doctors aren't supposed to do that, are they? 'Do you know who I am?' Why does he always ask me this? Is it because he knows I think he looks like my ex-husband? How can he know that's what I think?

He talks. I have no idea what he's saying. He seems pleased.

I have to ask him the question I dread and to which I know the answer.

Is it my fault? Did I bring this on myself? Am I the reason that I'm here in this hospital?

He shakes his head a lot and draws pictures in the air with his fingers, pictures that mean nothing. I catch the odd word here and there '. . . depuis naissance.' I've never known the difference between hereditary and congenital even in English, but I no longer make the effort to listen to his gentle but emphatic denial. It's too late. I've pushed myself too hard for years. It is my fault. 'Alors, Madame Lapotaire, pas du tout, absolument pas du tout.' I wish he wouldn't call me Madame Lapotaire: that's my mother's name. I'm Jane.

I have forgotten to which question 'absolutely not' is the answer, but I will not

13

forget it *is* my fault.

Lights snapped on. 'My eyes, my eyes!' I can't bear the light. Light is not my friend.

The electric bed is activated so that it comes slowly into a semi-upright position.The pain in my head comes back. One of my eyes is prised open by determined fingers and drops dropped in, which smart. Why are they putting drops into my eyes?

'Please be careful of my eyes. I've had two cataract operations . . .' I can't think what the French for 'cataract' is. It is a struggle to speak. The voice that comes out sounds thick and drugged. It doesn't sound like mine. It seems a superhuman task to speak French. I can't make my French sound like French. It is beyond me to make the effort to do the accent. I sound like my mother, speaking French with her noticeable English accent. My mother, drunk, slurring the words. My mother's voice is coming out of my body. It frightens me. She wished me harm when she was alive. Is all this her doing? It seems a preposterous idea, and the more preposterous it seems, the more convinced I become that it's true. I'm frightened of this voice.

'Madame Lapotaire!'

'Je ne suis pas *Madame* Lapotaire, je suis Jane,' I protest feebly. It seems important to me that they get it right. Insistent fingers force

14

the other eye open for more smarting drops. Two pairs of hands push me into an upright position. I shout as their hands, either side of me, force some of the needles and drips that are in my arms in deeper. But it's only my head I'm aware of. I scream, 'My head, my head!' I look down to where I feel the pinpricks. There are two thin arms, black and yellow with bruises from wrists to armpits. There is a body attached to them with no clothes on, wires and tubes and suction pads coming out of it at all angles. It means nothing to me.

Sitting up, my groin hurts on both sides. It hurts more than my head. Water trickles down over the breasts I can see if I lower my eyes, over the thin white body. It collects unpleasantly in my pubic hair and slowly insinuates itself either side of my vulva. 'Voilà, la petite toilette!' one of them says, in such a condescending manner I want to scream, 'If this is *la petite* what on earth is *la grande*!' I want to lash out at the face of the nurse who has spoken. I feel so invaded. Anger churns and rises up in me. I say the worst that I can think of: 'It's not surprising you had a revolution in this country.'

Greyness. How long I have lived in the greyness I don't know. I don't know morning from night in the greyness. I am not aware of days passing. Or nights.

15

Sometimes Ann's face swims into view on my left and sometimes it's not there. On the right side, to which I cannot turn easily but I'm not sure why, my son's face occasionally appears, smiling, attentive. I close my eyes, smiling. When I open them he's gone. Mostly I don't think, but when I do I think, Well, this is easy. This is fine, whatever it is.

CHAPTER TWO

Intensive Care?

'No, no, don't cut my nails! Don't! I need them long to stick the false ones to, for Callas!' The two nurses—they're always in twos—look at each other, then at me. I raise my left hand, which is not as easy as it seems with tubes and wires attached to it, and look at the nails. They are stubby and uneven, and there is blood under the quicks. Blood from where?

Ann sits on the bed and takes a nail file and scissors out of her manicure bag. 'No, Ann, no, I need them for Callas.' Why does no one listen to me? I'm so resentful of being helpless I'm dangerously near tears.

'I don't think you'll be doing Callas for a while . . .' she says gently.

'OK,' I say, rallying what I assume to be my most rational voice. 'I'll make a deal. I'll stay

16

here for a week.' I remember that there was a gap of a week between teaching in Paris and starting to re-rehearse Callas for the second eight weeks of the tour. That'll fit in nicely. So I have time. I have no idea where 'here' is.

Ann puts on her best professional nursing voice: 'I think it will be longer than that.'

A flood of enormous relief fills me. I am shocked by it. Callas has taken over my life since last May and I have been overjoyed to be walking in her shoes. But I am so tired. More tired than I have ever been. I sink back. No sadness, just relief. Ann goes on doing my nails. I let go of her hand. I let go of it all.

All is blue. Everything I can see is bright cobalt blue. How odd. It intrigues me, almost pleases me. But there's something else that's not quite right. It takes me a while to focus. I can see silhouettes. People are moving about the room but all I can see is their arms edged in blue, the outline of their heads and shoulders, all blue. They look like blue diagrams of themselves. The wall opposite is a rectangle of blue with nothing in the middle.

The bed is moving. Not in the undulating way it does when they press the button to raise or lower my head or feet, which isn't always unpleasant, as long as they don't raise my head too high. It makes me feel like I'm on a waterbed. But now the whole bed is moving.

These are different walls from the ones I usually look at, but it's dark and I can't quite see. The walls are moving. Am I in a lift? There are two men in the bright emerald green tunics of what I've assumed are the auxiliary nurses. The doctors, I think, are the ones who glide about in white. I struggle to sit up. I have suddenly an overpowering feeling of having had enough.

I reach down and, with some difficulty, pull the catheter out and say, 'I am going home.' All hell is let loose. 'Vous êtes folle!' Not asked as a question. 'You are crazy! You'll break your—' Then comes a French word I don't know. The catheter is pushed against my vagina. 'N'écartez pas les jambes! N'écartez pas les jambes!' My legs are held together. 'Madame Lapotaire, je vous en prie!' I think I'm struggling to get free of the hands that are holding my legs, but I don't seem to be moving. 'Non, non, laissez-là!' My legs swing apart. A laugh. 'On voit la marguerite!' More laughter. Mocking, unpleasant laughter.

I am naked now that the large J-cloth-like sheet is no longer covering me. My body is white and angular in the darkness of the lift, apart from all the usual tubes and suction pads that accompany me everywhere. All this time with no clothes on has inured me to any sense of embarrassment, but I am appalled that the description of my anus should be so ludicrous and so vivid. A daisy.

18

I want to explode with the injustice of what is happening to me. I am alone in this lift with these two men. I don't know what is happening, but I do know I am in hell.

Later, I complain about it to a nurse who makes all the right tut-tutting noises as yet another injection goes into my stomach. 'But, Madame,' I insist, 'it's disgusting, isn't it, to treat patients like that?' I notice there is a small round bluish bruise on my stomach from the injection the time before, from a nurse I don't like, and who I know doesn't like me. People's underlying attitudes seem so clear and obvious. She (the horrid nurse), I was convinced, applied extra pressure out of spite. 'Isn't it dreadful?' I persist, attempting to hang on to the incident in the lift.

'Oh, yes,' she says, and carries on twiddling the dials on the two machines that I can just see above my bed to the right. 'Mais oui.' She renews some of the needles in my arms.

I begin to feel I am in a world where all the usual modes of behaviour don't apply. 'What was that injection for?'

'Fleabitis.' I have no idea what that is. It doesn't sound clean. How on earth did I catch that in here?

The lift journey was real. Months later I learned that my brain had gone into spasm, which is not unusual, some days after the initial six-hour operation to clip the aneurysm and stem the bleed. Then they had to do an

19

angioplasty—insert a camera into my groin, up the femoral artery into the back of my neck and round to the front of my brain where the artery they had clipped was clamping down and blocking the flow of blood. This can cause a massive backlog of blood, which in turn provokes a massive stroke, then death. The camera turns into a balloon to keep the artery open. They did it twice.

That night—what night? Have I just been put back in my room from the lift? Is it night? I don't know. But I know I am angry. I am angry with God. I am angry with the entire world. I am so angry I want to shout. So shout, I think. I'm not sure I remember how. My head hurts. I want a wet face flannel on my head. Oh, why doesn't someone put a wet flannel on my head? It feels so comforting. It cools me down. Ann puts a cool wet flannel on my head when she's here. Why isn't she here? I feel six years old and helpless. I want my foster-mother, whom I called Gran, to make me better. Where is she? Where is my Gran? Somewhere in the smallest bit of my rational mind I know that she's been dead for fifteen years. But that's not fair. She should be here. This is serious, what I'm going through, whatever it is. I feel anger trickle back into the sadness. I am lit up by it. I don't believe in a personal God but I hear myself shout, 'Why did I have to go through all that in the lift? Why? Why?' Nobody answers but, then, I

20

don't expect anyone to. To be pushed about like a sack of worthlessness. I fume. I boil. I've never thought of myself as a particularly proud person, but something resembling pride is very disturbed. Yet I can do nothing. Or rather there is nothing that can be done.

I open my eyes. Is it morning or night? I don't know, but I know I'm in Croydon. There is a blonde ponytail belonging to a nurse I have never seen before, her back turned towards me. She is writing something on the vast white chart that takes up the entire wall opposite my bed. I think, When she turns round, she's going to speak to me in French. But I won't be fooled. I *know* I'm in Croydon. She turns round and says, 'Bonjour, Madame Lapotaire, vous allez mieux aujourd'hui?' See? Croydon! I think. I smile to myself inwardly. In some small way I feel I've won. They can't fool me.

Lights click on. In come two nurses. Oh, no, the trickling water again. I put my plan into action. The plan I thought of last time I was subjected to this ritual humiliation, but was too quickly, too firmly in the grip of the two previous nurses. 'Please, please, laissez-moi tranquille, j'ai mal à la tête.' Major brain surgery and I'm complaining of a headache. The room is empty. I can't believe my luck. I

21

feel fine. Rather well, in fact. No pain. Nothing. This is easy. Whatever it is.

Slowly I turn my head. It's hard to do. Not because of my head but because of the pain in the back of my neck. It's a burning stiffness, as if I've just finished a week of eight performances when all the tiredness and stress and exhaustion centre themselves in my neck. It's a very vulnerable area for most performers; most actors suffer stress in their necks, musicians too.

Above my head and slightly to the right are two television screens. I gaze, fascinated, at the variety of squiggles and graphs on them. I don't know how long it takes me to relate the patterns on these screens to my body. I don't really feel I have a body most of the time now. Just a head. Sometimes, like today, I have a neck. I want to play. I decide to hold my breath. I can't breathe very deep—all those cigarettes—but I aways managed to breathe deeply on stage. I manage to stop breathing out for a while. Don't breathe. Don't breathe. I concentrate on where I imagine my lungs to be. The back of my neck pounds with blood. I look up without moving my head. To my delight all the squiggles on the screens change shape. The breath bursts out of me and leaves me panting, feeling as if I have just run up the steepest hill with lead weights tied to me. It is beyond tired. I am all—what is it I am? Frailty, I think. That's what I am, frail. I've never

22

really thought about that word before. Before I can, I fall asleep.

Lights snapped on. Two nurse shapes approach. I am too tired to fight.

I am holding a piece of paper in my hand. It has bold, clear lettering on it done by a computer and a clear rectangle marked out in the shape of the paper with two lines. The message isn't important, but the name on it is. It comes from my ex-husband. So this, whatever it is, was worth it, then. With much difficulty I manoeuvre the piece of paper under the left side of my head as if to draw comfort from it, turn my head into it and drift. I feel strangely content.

When I next remember it, it isn't there.

When I ask Ann where it came from, she says it was with flowers, but I'm 'not allowed flowers in intensive care'. Oh, I'm not? Why?

'So where are they, then? The flowers?'

'I gave them to Dr Vinikoff.'

Well, of course that's right. Dr Vinikoff looks like my ex-husband.

I have a memory of tight, round, many-petalled flower-buds in deep rich reds and auburns, but I don't think I ever saw them.

Two nurses. Two emerald-green movements of busyness. 'Bonjour, Madame Lapotaire. Well, come on, say good morning. It's polite to reply when people say good morning to you,' or at least that's what I think she says. I can't hear. Whatever it is, it grates. I hate the French in their bossy mode. It's too close to home.

'I'm deaf,' I mutter. I catch them looking at each other in a silent, knowing way, as if I have just invented a new and particularly taxing problem. 'No, but I really am . . .' I have a hearing-aid, for goodness' sake, I think. Was I wearing it when . . .? I don't wear it all the time. Only when the need is so big it outweighs the vanity. Someone must have taken it out of my ear when . . . when . . . when what? When. I. Fell. Ann, probably. Suddenly it seems a worryingly intimate thing to have had done to me.

Ann put her finger into my ear and took that little pink plastic thing out. I worry that there may have been earwax in it. The lukewarm water trickles its familiar way down and over my breasts to collect in a puddle on the paper under me.

Ann sits and strokes my hand. It is very tender and loving. Sweet. I can't think what I have done to deserve all this attention but it's lovely. I don't want to go to sleep—she's only just got here. 'Go to sleep,' she says.

'But you've only just got here.'
'No, I came this morning too.'
'What morning?'
'Go to sleep,' she says again, so I do.

There's one who comes in who wears the green and has a black face. He often smiles at me. His badge says his name is Serge. I can read it clearly when he bends over me and does things to the needles in my arms and checks the tubes above my head. I know he speaks to me because I can see his lips move. I call him my *vert galant.* That makes his smile wide. My Green Knight.

My son is beside my bed again, smiling. I try to turn my head in his direction. His is the face I most want to see. 'When did you get here?' That sounds so normal, I think. 'Today,' he says. 'Last time I came it was Wednesday. I had to go back on Thursday, and they operated on you on the Friday.' My head spins with trying to make sense of all these days and can't.

'How long have I been in here, then?'

'Three weeks.'

'*Three weeks*?' It sounds nonsensical. All that time. 'You mean I haven't had a fag for *three weeks*?'

We laugh. I can smell smoke on his clothes.

I close my eyes to work out a joke about him unhooking the tubes and sticking a cigarette in my mouth. How I wish he didn't smoke. When I open my eyes he's gone.

Grey. Snap. The grey gets less dense. From behind my eyelids, which flicker in the light, I say, 'I have a headache. Please leave me alone. Laissez-moi tranquille un petit moment. Laissez-moi, s'il vous plaît.' I keep my eyes closed, smiling inwardly. I know this trick works.

'Oh, ça alors!' someone shouts very near my face. 'Madame, I'm sick of you interrupting my work. You're not the only one here! I have to get on with my work.'

The voice is rising on a crescendo, which seems to carry my brain with it. I'm in it before I have time to think. My voice is quicker than my brain, as it will be for several months to come. 'I'm not *your work*, I'm a person—avec des désirs, avec besoins.' It sounds so silly, but I'm convinced I can make her see it from my perspective even as I splutter for the words. 'Je suis une personne—' No, that's not correct French. 'Je suis quelqu'un—' don't forget the feminine version '—quelqu'*une* avec des besoins—'

'Et moi! J'ai besoin de faire mon travaille!' she screams into my face. Her eyes are huge behind her glasses. Her curly hair frames her

26

face as she stands with her back to the white board. It will go on. It will get worse. I know it. It's like some awful play. I feel I've seen it before or, more exactly, I know it, this sharp and ugly scene that's unfolding.

The other girl, with hennaed hair, makes some placatory gesture—I don't catch the name she calls the shouting one. Anyway, it makes no difference. The floodgates of anger and abuse and spitting resentment are unleashed at me. I think, this is, of course, absurd. I'm ill, aren't I? I'm the one who's ill.

The *vert galant* comes in. I think it will get better now. She doesn't stop. She goes on shouting. Somewhere I know that what she is saying is true. After all, it *is* my fault. I know he will stop this, though, the Green Knight. He will say it is wrong, what she's doing. On and on goes the voice. The Green Knight shrugs his shoulders and looks helpless. He picks up something and leaves the room.

What is it I have done? What is it that she hates about me? I am going to ask myself these questions many times in the months to come.

I see flowers. There is a picture of flowers on a wall. I must be in a different place. There was a lift. I can see what looks like a lobby. There are two men in black hats. They look like rabbis. It feels like Sunday. I slide into sleep, although it feels like sleep slides into me.

Ann sits by the side of my bed stroking my hand. I don't question why she is here. Of course, Ann is here. She's always here. She always sits on the left side. I don't question that either, but I discover later that it's to avoid my turning my head on to the right side. Sleep again engulfs me.

Ann stands at the foot of my bed and announces triumphantly, 'I'm wearing your underwear!' I can't think why she has taken to wearing my underwear. Later, much later, I'm reminded that we came prepared for three days and had to stay for five weeks. Ann, who won't speak even the little French she knows, braved the Métro every morning for an hour and back, and every evening for an hour and back, mostly to sit in silence, as she told me later, look at me and will me to live.

'I can't think of anyone I'd rather have wearing my underwear,' I say, uncomprehending but magnanimous.

My left side hurts. There is a dull ache coming from my left hip. 'Turn her,' I hear Ann say, in her best schoolmarm voice. Then she says it louder to make them understand. 'Turn her or she'll get bedsores.' I have no idea what the French for 'bedsore' is. Arms slide under my armpits and move me to another position. But there is no getting away from the pain in my side.

A white sheet is being twisted into a coil above me. A nurse at each end walks towards me, tightens the sheet across my chest and ties it to the rails at each side of the bed. I can't move my body. Smaller bits of sheet are attached to each of my wrists and then my feet. I can't move at all. I am aghast. 'This is—it's brutal what you're doing!' I splutter, not sounding at all as enraged as I feel. 'It's—it's *medieval!*'

As furious as I am, I'm quite pleased with this notion. It has no effect on them, however, or what they're doing. They go on talking as they tie and I have no idea of what they're saying, not just because I can't hear but I can't lip-read French. French mouths make different shapes when they form words. I boil at my feebleness, searching for a winning putdown. I come up with 'What was it that attracted you to this job? It can't have been gentleness, or caring for people.'

I spend considerable time working the fingers of my right hand around the bar towards the inside of my wrist, where I laboriously begin to unpick the knot. I have to do it mostly by feel as I cannot turn my head too far in that direction. Anyway, I can't see, the bed is in its down position, as it is most of the time. Slowly, with much effort to concentrate, I manage it, then untie my left hand.

Triumphant, I can't wait to tell my son how clever I've been. I've foiled their plans. When I do, hoping he'll be pleased that I'm so sparky, he just says quietly, 'Oh, Ma, you shouldn't have.'

I was never told it was bad for me to move.

CHAPTER THREE

On the Move

The Green Knight, Serge, puts a bottle of water, a purple velvet bag that smells of lavender, a photo of my son and me on his twenty-first birthday, a box of Kleenex, my bag of urine and a brown beret (a brown beret?) on top of my legs and pushes the bed into the corridor. I can feel the wheels rumbling beneath me. Ann is there. She walks beside the bed. Is she holding a tube? Where are all the other tubes? Serge seems happy. He is smiling. When Ann cocks her head round to look at me she is smiling too. There appears to be an air of celebration about this trundling along. I am not party to it.

The room in which we come to a halt has

orange blinds at the windows. They seem to be flapping gently; like the sails of a ship. The room, which has another bed in it, is diffused with a warm orange glow. Behind the blinds I might catch my first glimpse of daylight. It might be grey, but it will be daylight. I wish I could crane my neck to see but my neck burns when I try to move it. The bed is swivelled round against the wall. A few seconds later my head catches up with me. Or, to be more exact, much later my brain stops moving independently of my head. I close my eyes. The fatigue quells any more curiousity about where I am.

My throat is so dry. 'De l'eau, s'il vous plâit, de l'eau . . .' It's a plaintive voice. It is the voice of a little girl.
    Why won't they give me water?

It is dark behind the orange blinds. It must be night. Light is coming in from a window above the door. Outside, voices are chatting gaily. It can't be night. Where did the day go? The sound of heavy footsteps in the corridor. Wood on tiles? Up and down the footsteps go. My throat feels so sore, it must be an infection. I must ask them to give me something to make it better. 'Oh, please, bring some water.' I feel six years old and very near to tears. 'De l'eau, s'il vous plait, de l'eau . . .'

When the water comes it tastes like dark velvet silk, but it slides down the sides of my neck. I can't lift up my head to the cup. A nurse I've never seen before jerks the head of the bed up. This bed doesn't move smoothly like the other. My head is jarred. Even the mattress doesn't feel so soft. For some unaccountable reason my left side still feels sore at the hip. The nurse cradles my head so that I can reach the water. Her skin is cool where it touches the burning stiffness in the back of my neck. It's not so much the coolness, though, that comforts me. It is the closeness of another human being. I am filled with love for her. I smile and lap the water. I am content.

When the door to my room is left open I can see an old man in a room on the other side, slightly further down the corridor. He has a bandage on his head. I am shocked to see a bandage. It makes me think of wounds and cuts and blood, even though this bandage isn't wrapped all the way round his head. It's shaped like a skullcap, although it's further forward than the crown of his head. Hanging from it on a string is a matchbox that someone has painted green. When he moves his head, it swings like the tassel on a nightcap. I laugh.

'What day is it?' The question can't be addressed to me, so I make no attempt to answer it. 'On est quel jour aujourd'hui?' the voice insists. The question is so absurd I think I ought to laugh, but really I want to sink down again into the greyness.

My left arm keeps me from the greyness. It twitches involuntarily every few minutes. There is no pain in it, but I can't stop it moving. I am too tired to wonder.

'Mangez, Madame, mangez, ça vous apportera de la force.' I am being asked to eat. Why haven't they given me anything to eat before? I can't understand it, but willingly open my mouth to receive the whiteness from the little pot. It's cool and soothing and the grains of sugar in it intrigue my tongue. I want to eat and eat and eat.

The room is empty. I move my head slowly towards the right. There is a tall bedside table. I look at the picture of my son and the purple velvet bag next to it. I have no idea how they got here.

The orange blinds flap gently like the sails of a ship picking up a breeze. The softness of the sound lulls me away from the soreness in my throat. I drift to meet it.

'Please can I have some water?' I wake up, wondering who just spoke. I also wonder why my head hurts.

Between my thumb and the middle finger of the left hand I feel a perfectly round button, exactly the width of the pad on the tip of the finger. I know what it looks like. It's one of those pearl buttons, just slightly larger than a shirt button, but with four holes in it. I often sew them on my son's shirts. I can feel its slightly cold, translucent surface. When I raise my hand slowly to bring it into view, there's nothing there. But when I put my finger and thumb together again, the button comes back.

'De l'eau, s'il vous plâit, de l'eau,' I chant quietly to the empty room.

Inside this little pot in front of my face is a thick yellowish substance. A teaspoon of it comes towards me. I have no idea what it is and am reluctant to open my mouth. The spoon rests against my lips. I have an almost irresistible urge to blow a raspberry into it and send it all round the room. I feel like a naughty child. I like the feeling. I have to fight hard to overcome this. I am so tempted just to blow into the spoon. Somehow a little of the substance finds its way on to my tongue. It is the sweetest, sharpest of stewed apple. I slurp the rest off the spoon. 'More,' I order, rather peremptorily, forgetting to speak French. The tanginess of it is so acute it's just not possible. I want to hold the pot so I can gulp it down at my own speed, but I can't seem to galvanise my arms to take hold of it. Anyway, I can't spare the time. I want it and I want it now. I think, How ridiculous, only the French could conceive of putting stewed apple into a carton. I smother this ungrateful thought in case it makes the pot disappear.

'What day is it?' Someone I haven't seen before bustles in and smiles generally in my direction without responding to my question. 'De l'eau, s'il vous plaît, de l'eau.' I feel vaguely sick. 'Please can I have something for my throat? I think I have an infection.' A door is opened in what I thought was a blank white wall opposite the foot of the bed. The bustling disappears behind the door. I can hear moving about. I wait. I wait, determined to ask one of my unanswered questions again. The door remains closed. I forget to wait. Sleep seems so pressing.

'Quel jour est-il?' I'm embarrassed that I sound like I did in the lower third form. Such a simple phrase, I must have asked this question many times over the years, but now the words seem curiously lame and stilted. But at least I no longer hear my mother's rasping voice

35

coming out of my mouth.

'Il est toujours jeudi, Madame,' comes the curt response. The main door to the room shuts, snapping off the last word. What Thursday? I want to scream. But I also want to vomit.

My left arm twitches, turning in on itself as it does so. I try to stop it happening, but it's a bit like trying to stop hiccups. As soon as I'm sure that it's stopped, I forget about it. It's quite easy to forget about it. And then it comes back. I stare at my arm. The top skin is flaky and white, where it isn't blue, purple and yellow. But that's on the underside. There are no needles or tubes coming from the coloured patches but there's a plastic tap-like thing on the back of my hand covered in plaster. I wonder what it's for. I am overcome by such a weariness that even the twitching can't stop me sliding into sleep.

'And you mustn't get up without ringing this alarm bell.' I'm slumped in a semi-upright position. I have no idea how I got to be almost sitting. Getting up seems the most ridiculous notion. My head throbs, but I pay it no attention or perhaps it's just that my stomach, and what is going on there, takes all my concentration.

36

Ann is there, at the foot of the bed, smiling. 'Turn her,' she says, in her most commanding voice. 'Turn her.' Clacking clogs approach the bed. The footsteps sound like hammer taps on the lino. Arms envelop me and shift me off my left side on to my back. I want to go on rolling over to get away from the soreness and the nausea. Rolling over and over as we used to as children in the park. 'Non, non, Madame, ce n'est pas possible.' It is not possible to roll on to my right side. Why? I no longer care.

'You'll need this soon.' Ann puts a violently spotted navy blue and white dressing-gown on the bed. The spots shout and scream and jump out at me. They won't stay in their ranks. They begin to march in crazy divergent patterns. I have to close my eyes.

What day is it?

My stomach burns and churns. I feel nothing but nausea. Waves of it surge up from my gut. I can't remember ever having felt so sick. I want to vomit badly, but I know I won't. I suspect this is the kind of nausea that doesn't have an outcome even though my natural reaction is always to fight against it. I decide to ignore it. It's not at all pleasurable but at least I'm aware that I have a stomach. I am no longer just a head. I have a stomach. Then I wish this feeling of sickness would stop. My whole body is nausea. Time stretches.

'What day is it?'

A pouch of liquid is being changed above my head.

I want to scream the most violent abuse at the questioner. I say angrily, 'You know very well I don't have the vaguest idea and what's more *je m'en fous.*' I don't. I'm not playing their games and I don't give a fuck.

Now between my fingers there is a sheet of paper. I can feel the thinness of it. Its dry surface stretches out beyond the palm of my hand. I'm surprised that I can't hear it rustle when my arm turns in on itself towards my body. It's a regular turning, this twitch, like clockwork. I don't have a clock. If I did I could time it. But I don't even know what day it is. I get tired of holding the paper. My clenched hand aches. I open my fingers and let it go. I wait to hear it fall to the floor. I hear nothing.

Footsteps. Laughter. Footsteps. Talk. My stomach swirls and seethes.

A youngish face, framed with pretty blonde tendrils of hair, leans in towards me, shining a light into my drowsy eyes.

'Oh, I feel so sick . . .' I mutter to myself. 'J'ai de la nausée . . . j'ai très envie de vomir.'

'But, Madame, you should have said.' She clicks off the torch, pockets it and almost runs out of the room.

A syringe. Another needle points towards me. I offer my left arm gratefully. It tries to jerk itself free of her grasp, but she has tight hold of it. I catch my breath as if to explain my arm. 'Ça passera,' she says, in answer to my unasked question. I make out the words 'blood pressure' and 'automatic' as the needle bites deep into a vein. Instantly the sickness stops. My body is free of it. It is a miracle. I weep. Tears of relief.

'What day is it?'

I feel suspicious. They all ask this. Is this some kind of test? 'I have a sore throat. Please give me something for it. I ought to see a doctor . . . What day *is* it?'

'Le vingt-huit janvier.'

The door closes on the constant stream of chatter in the corridor. I go to sleep repeating, 'The vingt-huit janvier. The vingt-huit janvier.' I think. I should have been in Milton Keynes on the vingt-huit janvier. Playing Callas. I try to recall the text. I cannot think of one line of it. I pull the velvet bag of lavender from the table with my right hand and put it under my chin where it keeps my head at a comfortable angle. I stroke it. Where did it come from? The velvet is exquisitely soft under the pads of the tips of my fingers. I stroke it till sleep finds me.

'My head hurts.'

'I'll get you some painkillers.' Two red and white capsules are handed to me with a plastic beaker of water.

'What are they?'

'Paracetamol.'

I want to pee. No, worse, I want to crap. I don't know the grown-up version, so I say, 'Je veux faire caca,' not meeting the eyes of the nurses who are in the room. This six-year-old embarrasses me. Instantly a bed-pan appears, a white plastic thing, and I am lifted on to it. I scream with the pain. It digs into my lower back. The side of it catches the bedsore on my left hip. My head feels like an iron weight and I know that the burning muscles at the back of my neck aren't strong enough to support it. I worry that it will loll backwards. All this is not conducive to passing a motion as they say in the best medical circles. I pass, if that is the word for the pushing and the heaving, an amount that feels like it would put a fairly young rabbit to shame. The bedpan goes on digging in. I puff and pant with the discomfort. The door opens. People passing in the corridor can see me because I can see them. Ann appears.

'Oh, please, get me off, get me off. It hurts.' I feel pathetic, not embarrassed, just pathetic.

Efficiently Ann wipes my bottom, not

40

looking at me, and arms restore me to the hard mattress. 'Nothing's sacred,' she says, laughing as she disappears behind the small door. I want to laugh too. But somehow I can't. It is beyond me.

I like this nurse with the brown hair. She has a worn, kind face. 'What day is it?' I ask her slyly. 'On est quel jour aujourd'hui?'

'Mais, Madame, on est le deux.'

'Le deux de quoi?' The rhyme amuses me. *Deux de. Deux de.* I play with it in my throat, feeling the odd shape my lips make. 'Le deux de quoi?'

'Mais le deux février, Madame.'

February. February? I find this ludicrous, but deviousness is more important than ridicule.

'Could you write it on the board over there?' She turns to look at the whiteboard, which is covered with all sorts of medical squiggles and hieroglyphics, and is about to protest when I say, 'Write it at the top where no one can see. Write it in English.'

She is proud to be writing in English. In her best looping French writing she writes, as I spell it out for her, 'Wednesday 2 February 2000.' All the noughts make me want to laugh.

Later I make Ann laugh: 'Men on the bloody moon and they still haven't changed the shape of a bedpan.'

41

A menu is placed on the table that swivels across the bed. I look at it disbelievingly. Chicken. Rice. Salad. They seem alien words. I tick randomly without really relating the words to food. It's like a game with columns on bits of paper, but making the ticks seems laborious. It takes a lot of effort and time. I drift between the choices, unable to imagine what eating any of it will be like.

I want to pee. It's a strangely pleasant new feeling. No catheter. I wait. I'll wait till someone comes in . . .

Serge. When I open my eyes Serge is there. Serge has come to visit. He sits by the side of the bed like a proper visitor, not a hospital employee. We chat like old friends. He smiles and smiles at me, as if I have done something particularly pleasing to him. I can't think what it could be. I whisper to him conspiratorially that I want to pee and he becomes quite stern. 'You mustn't even try to sit up wthout help.'

Slowly and gently, he moves the bed-head into the upright position. 'Stay there, don't move.' I think this is absurd. Sitting up is easy if it weren't for this stupid pain in my groin.

Arms lever me off the many pillows. I am sitting upright. There are the familiar pains in my groin where my weight is in contact with the mattress, but where my head is I have no idea. It feels disconnected to the rest of my body. After much manoeuvring, the two nurses, now on the same side of the bed, facing me, are holding me in position. 'Move your legs now,' says one encouragingly. I look down at the two white, stick-like things that protrude from the J-cloth gown I have on, and think, Move your legs. Swing your legs over to the side of the bed. There is a faintly discernible trembling in the legs. I carry on looking at them dispassionately, as if they are not part of me. All the skin is flaking and peeling. Great strips of skin are loosely attached. Most of the surface looks like scurf. One of the nurses grabs my ankles and swings my legs towards her. They take me under the arms and lift me on to the floor. As my feet touch the cold, smooth surface of the floor, my legs crumble under me like pipe-cleaners. Were it not for the nurses I would have fallen. They half drag, half lift me towards the little door in the wall.

I am shaking as I sit on the loo. It is an uncontrollable tremor that is charging the whole of my body. Suddenly I have an acute sense of being alone. With no one else around my body has an awareness of itself. It is unusually quiet inside the lavatory, away from the clanging and talking in the hospital. Silence. I pull myself up using the washbasin. In the mirror is a face. It is grey. The eyes are sunken with purplish bruises around the sockets. The front of the right side of the head is shaved to the scalp, and there is a livid red

43

scar that runs from the middle of the forehead to the right ear. All the stitches that run across the angry red line are clearly distinguishable among the stubble of white hairs that are growing around them.

'J'ai terminé,' I say, like the child I feel, 'et j'ai mal à la tête.'

When Ann comes in bearing mango and avocado—a triumph for her to have shopped in French from a North African fruit stall near the Métro, even though she insists it consisted of a lot of judicious pointing—I cry. I cry as much as my head will allow.

'They should have warned you there was a mirror in there,' she says, 'or they should have covered it up.' Hard to explain that I'm not crying because what I've seen is ugly, though it is. I'm crying because now I know something serious must have happened. I have seen a scar.

They must use a drill to cut open the skull. Perhaps it smells like the burning chalky smell of teeth at the dentist. I shove the mango into my mouth with my hands, getting the stringy bits caught in my teeth, fumbling with sticky fingers to get hold of the ends and pull them out. I want to smother my face with the orange sweetness. To cry mango out of my eyes and breathe in the orange flesh. I want to cry till the whole of my head is quiet pulpy fruit.

I can't walk and I have a job to start in Denver in seven weeks. I must get moving. Why have I got a pain in my head?

I resent them coming in to get me out of bed to pee, so I begin not to ring the alarm bell in the night and try to get out of bed myself. It is a tricky, scary business. It takes me many manoeuvres just to sit up, even though I sleep almost vertical. Once up, I'm worried about falling and hitting my head. I move from bed edge to bed edge, to the foot of the other bed, but there's a few inches where I have to let go with my left hand in order to catch the door handle with my right and I'm in space unsupported except by my quivering shaky legs, which I can't and don't trust. I must walk again.

Ann walks me during the day. Down the corridor to the window at the end. We pass a man with a scar like mine, skulking in an alcove, smoking. The smoke smells acrid and turns my stomach. When I look at him, he looks away. I sniff at the open gap in the window like a dog. I lap the air. Outside, in the grey, is a formal French garden of the barest kind: low box hedge cut into square borders with nothing in the middle. But I yearn to be out there.

It can't be more than fifteen steps from my room to the window in the corridor. The return journey is a struggle where I count every one of them and hold on to Ann tightly, as my legs threaten to regress into woolly spirals. The hard mattress, even though it aggravates the bedsore, is the place I now most want to be in the world.

When I wake, Ann is busy washing up the knife and plastic box she brings from Gee's flat for the fruit relief. I was at Gee's flat, Ann still is. I watch her being busy. Ann loves being busy. She turns round to see me watching her. I smile. She smiles back. 'Little treasure.' She calls me that when she's pleased with me. We've only been friends for five years. She turns to look at me and appraise the situation. She neatens the sheets, her erstwhile nursing training coming to the fore; she clucks approvingly on checking the corners, straightens up, looks at me again and says, 'Hell and back!' There is an air of triumph in the room. Triumph in which I have had no part. 'I thought you were a goner, girl. Well, we all did. I sat by that bed day after day and I willed you to live.' She says it with a lot of emotion. A lot of emotion for her. I don't know whether to be happy or sad. 'I willed you to live. I thought, I lost Jamie, but I'm not losing you.'

I am struck by an undeniable rush of acute discomfort. I don't know why, but this seems terribly wrong. Jamie was her lover of fifteen years. She shouldn't have said that. I've only

46

known her for five years. But that's not it. It's not the length of time that's wrong. I look away.

'What's the date?'

I sneak a look up at the whiteboard and try to count on my fingers how many coffee trolleys have been round. 'February the third,' I answer proudly. 'And I want to go home. I want to go to England.'

'Why?'

'That's my home. That's where I live.'

'Why?'

'I'm English.' How odd to be in France saying I'm English, when I'm normally in England saying I'm French. There is something topsy-turvy about this world.

Scissors on my scalp. The clip-clip of sharp steel blades is disconcerting. It is very loud, so close to my good ear.

'What are you doing?'

'Hygiene,' comes the terse reply. More snip-snip-snipping.

'What are you doing?'

'Don't move your head.'

I don't move my head, though the effort of keeping it still makes the muscles in my neck burn and burn.

'What?'

'Sssh. Tidying you up.'

The old man in the room opposite has lots of visitors. He's now progressed to staggering about the room with the help of many arms and much loud encouragement that seems to have a *provençale* twang to it. The old lady who comes every day, who looks as frail as he is, must be his wife.

'You could have ended up in a wheelchair, Ma, or been paralysed or unable to speak.'

'Could I?'

'Oh, yes.' He says it with an air of wonder and I detect a subtle thread of praise. But what he says has no meaning for me. What have I done? I know he's pleased, because he strokes my head gently, sitting in his usual position on the right side of the bed, smoothing the hair that's left near the scar, which I can now picture. I want him never to stop. But soon he has to get the train at the Gare du Nord. It is near the hospital. I don't know the Gare du Nord, and I don't know the hospital, and I don't know when I will see him next. I feel flooded with sadness, but the love that I feel in his touch stops me crying. I mustn't cry, I'm the mother, I must be strong.

What day is it?

They get me out of bed, so it must be

morning, and I fall asleep in the chair. I find that shocking. I never fall asleep in chairs. Why am I so tired? I've only just been lifted out of bed. It seems such a long wait for the rattling trolley with the scalding hot coffee and *biscottes* that I load with all the jam from the little plastic squares that are such trouble to open. My head drops forward till the burning in my neck jerks me awake. I have dribbled on to the jumping blue and white spots. Gooseberry, redcurrant, such odd choices for breakfast jams. I long for marmalade, but I daren't think of that: it reminds me of home. Home. But I'm not going home. I have a nine-month job in Denver. I have to pack up my home for nine months and go to Denver. I loathe the largeness of the spots on this dressing-gown. I can't stop them moving.

The door opens and a man in a white coat, whose face I've seen before, walks in, followed by another man in a white coat whom I don't know. They walk to the far side of the room. Then a green uniform, followed by another green uniform, and another and another . . . The door is shut and there is silence. I am aware that they are all looking at me. I look back at them. Anger rises in my throat. 'What do you want?'

The first man in the white coat says, 'We've come to see how you are.'

I want to say, 'Well, you've got a bloody funny way of showing it,' except I'm not at all amused. I am seething. The anger is like a lump in my chest now, which makes me catch my breath and breathe hard. 'I'm fine,' I say curtly. I think how stupid French is—I'm going well, *je vais bien.* I'm not going anywhere.

The silence is renewed.

'Don't you think it's a little bit . . .' I want to say 'insensitive', but I can't think of the word in French so I say '. . . rude to just stand there and stare?'

'Well, you're an actress, aren't you?' says the first white coat.

I cannot believe I am hearing this. 'Yes, but I'm not working. You're not always on duty either, are you?'

I do not recognise the woman who just spoke.

They seem astonished too, but I detect that their astonishment is tinged with a smug collective pride. I am livid. I want to shout and bash things. But there is a pain in my head.

They file out.

Ann has brought me a clock, so now I know the difference between the grey of a winter morning and the identical grey that I catch in strips under the blind that heralds a winter evening. Anyway, the talk in the corridor is louder at night.

Ann says, 'Your friend David turned up. At the hospital door.' She sounds almost offended.

'Yes, he comes to Paris a lot. He has a daughter who lives here . . .'

'I sent him away.' She begins to cut up the blessedly soothing mango and avocado into cubes, which I will stuff into my mouth, after my half-crawl, half-lurch to the loo in the middle of the night. It makes me feel deliciously wicked, eating when everyone else is sleeping, apart from the night staff laughing and talking in the corridor.

'And Patricia rang from London to say she has her case packed and can come to Paris any day. I said, "No, no visitors."' She smiles, knowing that she has done right, that she is protecting me. I know I have been very ill. Am. Ill. I suppose I don't want people to see me with all those tubes and drips, do I? She smiles again and settles down to do my nails. She is right, isn't she? I look away. I was, am, too ill to care. I cannot make a decision. It is beyond me. I escape into sleep.

A telephone is brought into my room. There is much bustle and import.

'Your sister.' Ann leaps out of her chair. 'How did she get to know you're in here? No one is supposed to say—' Ann looks cross. She knows that my half-sister and I don't get on at the best of times. We never lived together as children. She lived with the Lapotaires in

51

North Africa and I lived with Gran in Ipswich. We have nothing in common, and even when I'm well I hate the phone. Besides, I realise I'm not strong enough to hold it, even to my bad ear. My good ear is where the end of the scar now is.

'Please take it away. I don't want it.'

The nurse bends down to plug in the phone beside my bed.

'I don't want it!'

Ann stands by, helpless to intervene in French.

Now I'm getting cross and it hurts.

Ann looks concerned.

'You mustn't get upset.'

Too late.

'I don't want the telephone in here.' I'm dangerously near shouting. 'Je ne veux pas le téléphone!'

The nurse looks up at me, 'But it's your sister.'

'She's not my sister, she's my half-sister.' I realise how ridiculous an answer this sounds. Explaining the family's chequered divergence seems as daunting a mountain of effort as explaining to my half-sister what has happened to me. Anyway, I don't know what has happened to me. Ann keeps telling me the bits between the blacknesses but I can't seem to retain them, or the order they came in. My head is now throbbing and there are pains in my chest. Pains that I recognise of old as exhaustion.

'Enlevez-le!' The nurse stands up slowly with the unplugged telephone in her hand. She looks at me quizzically. This is the second time it has happened. I am an odd animal. Someone who doesn't want to speak on the phone. Ann rinses the flannel she has brought me in cold water and puts it on my head.

When I open my eyes there's a copy of *Hello!* magazine just inches from my face. Ann chuckles. 'You can imagine how far I had to traipse through Paris to get this!'

Delight. Glamorous, frivolous, escape trash. I grab it.

'Not for *now*,' Ann says, 'for later, when you've had a chance to . . .' I can hear that she doesn't want to mention the recent upset '. . . to recover. Oh, and there's this.' She hands over an envelope with beautiful neat writing that I recognise.

'Oh, it's from Paul Jesson! He has such beautiful handwriting.' She smiles. I smile back.

'Not a lot wrong with you,' she says maternally.

One day I pluck up courage to ask for another bowl of coffee from the breakfast trolley. Its hot syrupy sweetness—I put all my packets of sugar into it—is the highlight of the beginning of the day. They seem to wake me up at dawn to take my blood pressure. There's only a weak tremor in the left arm now. They give me jabs and shine lights into my eyes and haul me into a different position in the bed, but I usually drift back to sleep after the assault.

I'm only ever allowed one cup of coffee. Today I am about to ask for two. I am prepared for all sorts of outraged reactions and refusals. 'Mais oui, certainement, Madame,' says the trolley lady, so kindly I am awash with tears that sting my throat. I swallow them down with the sweetness. The coffee has the desired effect, although perhaps not as thoroughly as I could've wished. After my usual half lurch, half crawl to the bathroom, I sit on the loo holding my head against the pain of straining; I think wryly that, however dramatic or romantic the illness, it all boils down to sitting on a loo praying for help with constipation.

A pile of pills is thrust into my lap. I look at them, uncomprehending. 'What are these?'

'These are your tablets.'

'What are they for?'

'There's the yellow ones three times a day, the pink one at night, and the two white ones also at night.' These I recognise, I took them before—*before*—in England, one for the gut, the other for the bladder. 'The other small

54

white ones are first thing in the morning. They're anti depressants—you said you were feeling depressed yesterday.'

What was yesterday? When was it?

'Did I?'

'Yes.'

'Well, I was.' Hard to admit.

'Depressed?' There's a note of accusation in the voice—not surprising: this is the nurse who gives me the injection in my stomach for phlebitis, which, I now know, is to prevent the collapse of all the veins in the body. She gives it to me with evident relish. I took to musing that maybe she'd had an English boyfriend who'd jilted her, or some other hatred of the English, and I was carrying the can, or at least my stomach was. There is still a bluish-yellow circle near my navel from the jab she gave me several days ago. The other daily shots don't show.

Yes, I was depressed. Am. I want to go home.

'The red and white ones—'

'Are painkillers, that I know. They don't seem to be very strong.' I don't mean to sound complaining but I do. 'Not very strong . . .' I trail off weakly. What I mean is, not strong enough. I can buy paracetamol over the counter at the chemist, for Christ's sake.

'Well, not after a morphine drip. After morphine nothing is.'

Morphine. Christ. I must have been ill. Am.

'And the yellow ones?'

'They're anti-epilepsy.'

'Epilepsy?'

'Yes, often brain surgery causes epilepsy.'

I push the pills aside and say, 'You'll have to give them to me as you always do. I can't remember all that, I just can't.'

A tall gentle black woman has come to occupy the other bed. She is regal and contained as she slowly unpacks her belongings. She has three huge sons who take it in turns to sit by her. She sleeps most of the rest of the time. We talk desultorily. She knows she has an aneurysm. She went to her doctor complaining of bad headaches and they scanned her head and found it. Momentarily, I regret all the painkillers taken for what I thought were headaches from a bad back. Even though she doesn't know for sure when her operation is I feel for her—she's aware that she's going to have her head drilled open. I think I was lucky: there's a lot to be said for just falling down.

'Vous allez mieux, Madame?' The quiet serenity of Dr Vinikoff alights on my bed. How curious. He doesn't look at all like my ex-husband now. He is balding, plumper in the face, and exudes peace. I think, this man has touched my brain, I can't quite get my mind round that one either, but the thought that he saved my life is a huge, stark fact.

I don't know how to begin to say, 'Thank

you, thank you for my life, thank you for saving me . . . thank you for giving me another chance.' It all sounds such melodramatic nonsense. This is the man who shaved my head himself before he operated, so that only the minimum of hair was taken off. How French.

'Dr Vinikoff, why has my hair gone white?' I point to the area around the scar. (The rest of it is dyed Maria Callas brown.) 'Is it the shock of what's happened to me?'

For a few seconds his serious, kindly face is troubled and preoccupied while he searches for an answer. I can't let it go on too long. I'm bubbling, like a child, with the fun of it. 'It's a joke! I haven't been to the hairdresser to get my roots done!' Only when I repeat, 'It's a joke, it's a joke,' does he allow himself to smile.

The hairdresser, I think. The real world. The idea fills me with fear. I say, 'When can I go home?'

'After the weekend, I think,' he says cautiously, 'but we have to talk about the other aneurysm first.'

Another one.

Another potential brain bomb.

I am devastated.

A bunch of exquisite flowers arrives. Flowers I have to sign for. The pen feels oddly long in my hand. I sign my name with a signature I don't recognise. The flowers are tight, cream and pale green, many-petalled buds of something I have never seen before. I marvel at them, and spend long minutes drinking them in from where they stand proudly on the table opposite my bed. They make me think of spring. A time of hope. They are from the President of the Royal Shakespeare Company.

Ann has brought in pyjamas, sent from London by Lise, the friend who works looking after my house and mail when I'm away. They're only British Home Stores tartan, they're old and washed-worn, but they're from home. I want to bury my face in them and sniff and sniff the smell of home. Ann helps me put them on. A flurry of flaking skin falls from my arms as I pull on the top. I try to put the bottoms on as I'm used to, standing on one leg at a time, but the room starts to swim and I lurch towards Ann, who grabs me even tighter. 'Sit down! You'll have to sit down to do the legs.' Like an old woman, I think. Old women sit down to put on their tights and trousers. I've been expecting 'people' to say, 'But you're so *young* to have had a . . .' whatever it is I've had, but no one has. I remember that I have to start work in Denver in two months. Friends will be staying in my London home for the nine months I'm away.

The red tartan of my p.j.'s and the white

spots of Ann's dressing-gown go to war on my trembling body; the clashing patterns jar my head and offend my sense of taste. But Ann has been kindness itself so I say nothing about the riotous dressing-gown. Ann's had a lot to deal with. She has stayed at Gee's flat all this time, Gee whom both of us barely know. Gee pops in occasionally, wearing a dashing, large-brimmed hat and a loden-green coat, which is pleasing to look at. Her soft American drawl is gentle on my ears, even when she speaks her fluent French. All my needs or queries go via Ann to her, and she deals with them. Gee is the kind of woman who deals with things. As does Ann. They are a powerful combo.

Gee did suggest, on one flying visit, bringing in a camera to Intensive Care and taking pictures of me, so that I could see later what I looked like. Ann said, 'No,' in that quiet, firm way she has, which means no and, what's more, that no further discussion will be brooked.

I insist today, in spite of Ann's reluctance, on walking the corridor twice. For once I'm hardly interested in what's going on on the other side of the window. Today I want to go the distance, and then some. I make sure the nurses see me. I say to Ann, loudly enough for any nurse who speaks English to hear as we make our slow, stately, shaky way down the corridor, 'I'm going home soon.'

'To Holly Cottage,' says Ann quietly. Holly

Cottage is where Ann lives. It has no holly.

A huge basket of fruit arrives. Mounds of fruit.
More fruit than I have ever seen in one basket.
Bananas, apples, oranges, pears, kiwi fruit,
dried apricots and figs. It is from the British
ambassador in Paris. I am impressed. How
kind. I suppose it's his job to cherish Brits who
fall by the wayside in Paris. I feel very
important. I pounce on the figs like a woman
demented, until Ann stops me scoffing the lot
in one go by removing them from my grasp.

On one of the rare occasions that my friend
in the next bed isn't sleeping, I offer her some
fruit. She shakes her head sadly. How stupid of
me. Of course she can't eat: she's still waiting
for her operation. When she uncurls her tall
frame and wanders over, in all her Senegalese
grace, to admire the mound, she asks me
who the fruit is from. I say, 'L'ambassade
Brittanique à Paris.' She gives me a decidedly
disbelieving look.

I return to reading *The Spy Wore Red*, which
Ann has brought me from Gee's library. I have
never read a spy book in my life. But I've
already devoured *Bella Tuscany* and *A House
in Tuscany*, which Ann had with her as she's
off to Tuscany later in the year. Ann's copies
of the *Spectator* have also served their turn.
With much despising on my part. But my avid
appetite for anything to read—an escape I

always turned to as a child—has been somewhat modified by my reluctance to rise to the largely right-wing diatribes of its regular contributors, so Ann has deemed the spy book more suitable light reading. I think it's stuff and nonsense. But I must not say so.

I dream a vivid dream. There is a man with a beard and glasses who lives in a house full of books, next to a church. It is St Michael. He asks me to marry him. The bizarreness of the dream unsettles me. It stays with me for a long time. What have they done to my brain?

Torchlight in the eyes. I blink away from it. The manual blood-pressure machine pumps away at my left arm. I don't care.

'On est quel jour aujourd'hui?' I sneak a glance at the whiteboard.

'Today is the fourth of February and I am going home.'

I am triumphant. The nurse looks up at me. It is obvious she hasn't been told. I am going home, aren't I? My triumph is only momentarily dimmed. Ann has already cleared most of the bedside table. There's little left on it. That must be proof. I pick up the purple velvet bag with my right hand, put it on my belly and stroke it. I look at the photo of my son. I wish he were here on this day. The day I'm going home. Well, actually, we're going to Gee's flat for a few days, so that I can get used to . . . so that I can . . . what was the phrase Ann used? 'Find my feet.' Find my feet in Paris before going to Holly Cottage.

Holly Cottage. We speak it like a mantra, Ann and I. The cure for all ills. Holly Cottage. Warwickshire. Holly Cottage. Spring.

I say goodbye to my friend. My room mate. I never did know her name. She told me but I couldn't hear. She spoke so softly, maybe, because of the pain in her head. We kiss with all the closeness of accomplices. I'm glad she doesn't really know what's in store. I wish her luck. Ann has packed some of the fruit, but the rest I say we're leaving for her. She thanks me and says, 'Mais les fleurs? Vous prenez sûrement les fleurs? Elles sont tellement belles.'

'Oui, elles sont belles.' Gently I finger the buds, which have opened just a little in the warmth of the room. 'Elles viennent du Prince de Galles.' As I pick them up and turn to take Ann's arm, I catch a distinct look of concern in the woman's watery black eyes, which I have no trouble interpreting. She is thinking, After I've had this operation will I end up as mad as her?

We have to pass through the decompression chamber of Dr V's office first. I am wearing the clothes I wore that day—the day I . . . that day: 11 January. Ann says we've been here five weeks. Today is 4 February. My mind goes into a time bend. My jeans feel thick and bulky and oddly stiff. But shoes feel oddest of all. I feel as if I am walking in two large cardboard boxes that have minds of their own. Without Ann's arm, I would be veering all over the place on the shiny, bewildering, patterned floor. I sit thankfully, at last, in a chair, encased in my nylon fur coat, while Gee, who I am surprised to see, comes in with us. I remonstrate and insist I can manage alone. After all, I'm better, aren't I? I'm going home. All is French efficiency and order in the outside room where we wait and whisper. I want to scream, 'I'm not a child!' But if I did, that would be proof that I am. Ann confirms that Gee is coming in with us, so all three of us troop into the inner office. It is as if I am being chaperoned by two maiden aunts. Gee translates into English for Ann what Dr Vinikoff is saying. No one looks at me.

I feel as if they are all talking about someone who isn't present. Resentment bubbles under the black fur. Then an overwash of guilt that I feel such resentment. The conversation between Gee and Dr Vinikoff is full of medical words that mean nothing to me. There are grey and black pictures that look like enlarged negatives hanging on clips by an illuminated board. They are of my brain. I am almost afraid to look. My gaze avoids that end of the room. I have to come back for another scan soon. 'March,' he says, 'late March.'

'But I'll be in Denver.'

There is a silence in the room. Why doesn't someone speak? It's because of Denver that I pushed myself to walk so soon.

'Early March?' I offer.

A date is arranged between the three of them.

'The second aneurysm?' That's from Ann— Gee translates.

Dr Vinikoff waves his hands dismissively in the air, and approaches me with one of the plates. I think I understand something about three centimetres and eleven centimetres. 'They won't operate until it's bigger,' says Gee.

I cannot countenance going through all that again. Somehow it gets mangled in my head and my whole being is submerged in fury with Ann for having brought the subject up. I must get out. If only I could get out of here everything would be all right. 'Things' would go on as before. I am hot with impatience. Ann sees my discomfort and comes over to help me off with my coat. She is so kind and thoughtful. I hate myself.

More talk that I don't understand, or register, or care about, between Ann and Gee, between Gee and the doctor. I hear my foster-mother's voice:

> Don't Care was made to care
> Don't Care was hung,
> Don't Care was put in a pot
> And stewed till he was done.

My real mother didn't care and look what happened to her.

I decide I will bring a present for Dr Vinikoff when I come back. What present could be adequate thanks for the saving of a life?

'You are very lucky, Madame Lapotaire.'

'Yes,' I say, feeling chastised. 'Jane,' I say. I pluck up my courage and add, 'Thanks to you.' He looks away modestly.

'Do you smoke?'

'Yes.'

'If you smoke you'll die. Smoking distends the arteries in the brain. The titanium clip—'

Rudely I interrupt him and say, 'I'm an ex-smoker.' There is a hint of a smile on his face.

I suddenly feel so overwhelmingly tired that I want to cry. Can't cry. Mustn't cry. They won't let you out if you cry. The more insistent my mother became in the asylum, the less they listened. I stand up shakily with Ann's help. She has her hands full of pieces of paper—prescriptions for pills that Gee will collect from the hospital pharmacy before we leave. What would I have done without these two women? I feel grateful, elated, resentful, fearful, relieved, hopeful—and utterly helpless.

CHAPTER FOUR

Up and Out in Paris

We walk from the lift, where I'd clutched Ann tight as my body descended but my head hadn't, down a long marbled corridor with columns that flit by at the edge of my vision towards The Outside. People pass by, surprising me by not knowing how jubilant I am, or how unsettled their passing is making me. There's a rack of cards outside a gift shop. Its colours shout and clamour for attention. Someone spins it as we approach and my head goes with it. I have to look away. At last I am in it, The Outside. The air is chill. It smacks me in the face. I gasp to take it in. I feel it travel into my lungs where it settles as an icy rawness. I look up to the sky, as much as my neck will allow, and soar into the glorious emptiness of it.

A group of young people are talking aimlessly nearby. One is wearing a white coat and has a stethoscope round her neck. I want to congratulate her for working in such a brilliant hospital, a hospital that has saved my life. I want to shout at them, 'I'm alive, I'm alive,' but instead, at Ann's bidding, 'Sit!' I readily sit down on a stone bench to recover from the fifty-yard walk. The cold of the stone

66

and the dampness of the day seep into my quivering body with alarming speed. I can't keep still. I am very cold. To my right is the only strip of Parisian street, complete with the maroon awning of a café, that has been visible to me from the hospital window. I look at it with love. Memories of Lapotaire, my stepfather, drinking pastis, watching me gorge on *milles feuilles* under his pleased gaze, flood back. I want to tell him too, 'I am alive. French surgeons saved my life!' But he has been in the Cimitière de Thiais for twenty-two years. Somehow I know he knows. Perhaps better than I do. I am alive. It is a phrase I have begun repeating to myself as if the repetition will help it become more real. As an idea, a fact, I know it is true; as an experience it means nothing yet. At all. I am alive. I am alive. As if what happened, happened to someone else; which of course it did.

Gee arrives with the car at the main entrance to take us back to her flat. The flat we had stayed in a lifetime ago, for one night, in another life. I turn round gingerly to take one last glance at the pleasing symmetry of the huge rectangle of hospital building, laced with doors, arches and orange blinds. Its grey roof, edged with horseshoe-shaped attic windows, catches the only remaining glint of winter light.

I wonder how it must have looked to my son each time he came in through those huge metal gates from the train, not knowing whether his mother was alive or dead. 'What's it called again, Ann?'

'Lariboisière.' Said with a weary familiarity.

'Lariboisière,' I murmur to myself. Strange barely to know the name of a place where I have spent over a month of my life—such a decisive month. 'Hôpital Lariboisière,' I say quietly, almost touching the scar, well protected from the winter cold and gawping eyes, under my blue wool hat, and quieter, 'Lariboisière, merci pour la vie.' I turn on the ever-present proffered arm to walk towards the street.

I'd thought I would feel safer in the back seat. With Gee and Ann in the front talking below the level I can hear, I recall again how like a child I feel. I snuggle into my coat with one hand on my chest and the other on my diaphragm. That gives me a shred of comfort and protection.

Cars, people, horns, engines, neon lights, traffic lights, pedestrians, cyclists, advertisements, taxis, shop windows, lamp-posts, pigeons, posters, sacks of garbage, rows of fruit, vegetables, rails of clothes, colours, dots, squares, stripes, lights, all converge and rush pell-mell into a bleary confusion as I squeeze my eyes tight shut against the world I have so wanted to see. It overwhelms my eyes and batters at my brain. It is all so vivid. So acute. I hold on to the car door as we take a cobbled street corner seemingly fast, bumping and turning. My brain bumps but it takes its own time to turn. I can feel it inside my head. It is most strange.

The elegant curve of the thirties staircase sweeps me up into it. It is quite beautiful. Why did I never notice it before? Its rising swoop threatens to lift me off my feet. I put out a hand for Ann. The clanking of the little wooden doors to the lift makes me flinch. My stomach rises into my throat with each successive floor that we climb. It will never stop. At last I step gingerly over the gap between the lift and the floor into the lobby of Gee's fine home. A little dog is running up and down. It is so pleased to see her. It's wagging its tail and its whole body is squirming with delight. I can feel its energy. It is palpable.

'Gee,' I say, 'Gee, your little dog is so pleased to see you! He's beside himself with joy!'

Gee stops in her tracks and turns sharply to look at me. 'My little dog died years ago.' There is a silence full of unasked questions.

'Oh, I know he's dead but he's still pleased to see you.' My raw brain is picking up the unseen dog's energy patterns. 'He's running up and down—'

Ann interrupts: 'That's enough, young lady. Bed!'

They look at me, still questioning, and I look back at them.

The sight of my suitcase, where I'd left it in the room I slept in all those weeks ago, makes my heart heave. I bend down to open it and look at the things inside. It's only an old Marks & Spencer's job but it seems redolent with all the yearning for home that's brimming over in my raw chest. I try to stand up, for fear that Ann will come in and tick me off for getting upset, and I can't. My legs simply will not support the weight of my body and propel it into an upright position. I try again. I have always been able to force my body into doing what I want it to do. I could always harness something. Not now.

'Ann,' I call as gently as I can, for fear of alarming her, turning my increasingly stiff neck into the direction of her bedroom. Within seconds she is in my room, white-faced and wondering. 'I can't stand up! I just can't get my legs to stand me up.'

She looks relieved that that's all it is. 'Well, are you surprised after three and a half weeks in Intensive Care?' Carefully, with her arms under my armpits, she hauls me into a standing position. 'What were you doing down there anyway?'

I can't say, 'Stroking my suitcase, touching my things.' She'll think I'm mad. My son would understand. But he isn't here. He can't be here. He's working. My legs feel like lead. Ann helps me undress. I sink gratefully into a proper bed. Ann leaves the door ajar. I cry quietly into my hands so that she can't hear, or worry. Within seconds my body is heaving with great shattering sobs, the kind of sobs that come from a long build-up. I'm catching my breath with the staccato force of them. They expel themselves in ever-diminishing waves, then renew themselves in the next onslaught. These yelps have been triggered by a few quiet tears and come from a very deep place somewhere in the body. This body which is no part of me.

I spend a long time when I wake, playing with the headscarf that Ann has thoughtfully put out. I didn't know what it was for at first. She brought it into the hospital where I didn't really bother with it. We all knew why we were in that ward, it was a question of 'Oh, his scar is at the base of his skull, her scar is above her ear.' And there weren't, except for the lavatories, any mirrors. Or people to be shocked. But here, I suppose, I have to spare people the sight of the scar. It is still black and angry in places but there is a good scab, which is healing along the line of the cut with its many transverse stitches. I spend too long with my arms above my head: the bedroom begins to spin and I have to sit down.

Lise, who used to babysit my son and now

looks after my things in London while I'm away, phones. She cries. I cry. London feels a bit more real than I can handle. My son phones and I cry. I have trouble holding the telephone. I can't hold it for long. My good ear is too near the scar. The left ear is deaf and, anyway, the left hand doesn't seem to want to grip. Ann keeps a wary eye on me from the kitchen and I have several warnings about not getting upset or wearing myself out. After eight years of living alone it feels like such a luxury having someone caring about how I feel.

I wander shakily through the palatial flat. Past the exquisite wood panelling that was installed here from a seventeenth-century château, past the woman in her satin-corseted dress reading quietly in the alcove of a little reading room off to the side, wobbling my way into the airy circular salon at the end. There, encouraged out on to the balcony, I spy the ever-effervescent Eiffel Tower still displaying her pink fizzing skirt. I hang on to the railings for fear of plunging over, always a ready fear but now an alarmingly real possibility. I lurch, or feel as if I do, although I don't seem to have moved my feet. My head seems to have flown off among the rooftops and the *garconnières*. I lurch again and have to be led inside. I sink into an armchair whose depth I misjudge, it is so soft and deep. I don't want to sit next to anyone. Not even Gee's friends on the sofa, one of whom is a particularly gentle and quiet man, William, a doctor who speaks English with the soft American burr he picked up while training in the States. I don't want anyone too near. The armchair surrounds me comfortingly. It feels like a hug. I never want to move.

The conversation flows back and forth in English and French, except for Ann, whose French still has her tongue-tied, and Bernard, Gee's lover who can't or won't speak English. The talk seems fast. It seems to have a note of celebration about it. Ann and I met all these people the night before I . . . all those weeks ago, so the evening has something of the air of a reunion about it too. The conversation switches from sofa to chair, to the other armchair, to stool, from chair to sofa—I realise I'm turning my neck in the direction of whoever's talking but not following a word. I'm not sure what the laughter is about. I think it might be about me. There are lots of smiles in my direction, looks of approval. I don't know what's going on. I can't follow so I bow out. But the voices go on jangling in my head. I suspect Bernard senses this, as he turns to me occasionally, assuring me that now I must have what I like, do what I want, that I have been magnificent. William, the charming doctor, confirms Bernard's opinion. The praise makes me feel shy—I wallow in every second of it, but I wish I knew what it is that I have done.

Waves of time later I tell them what I want to do. I want to take Ann up and show her Montmartre, all the lights of Paris from the top of the hill; then we'll have a dinner somewhere special, like the Breton restaurant that my stepfather knew. We'll have real Breton pancakes made on a griddle by the old gran'mère in the corner, from buckwheat flour, then we'll walk down, then we'll . . . More laughter.

'Maybe not tonight,' says William kindly, and adds that if there's anything I want to know about my 'condition' he'd be only too happy to answer my questions. What could I possibly want to know? I think. I'm out of hospital. I'm all right. Everything's all right.

Ann says I can't drink alcohol, but I keep an ever-watchful eye and mentally grudge every mouthful that everyone else takes. I glower from behind my lowered eyes and sip my apple juice. I can't smoke either, hard with drinks being handed out, hard anyway. 'It's hard not smoking.'

'No, it's not,' says Ann, from the other side of the room.

'*You* don't know,' I retort outraged. 'You've never smoked.' My voice rises and gets louder. 'No one who's never smoked can possibly know how hard it is.'

'Sssh,' says Ann. I want to slap her.

As I can't drink wine, dinner loses that particular dimension of attraction, but I fall on

74

the food with such relish that I am unaware that the speed with which I am shovelling it down might cause offence to Gee's guests till Ann gives me several veiled but meaningful looks. I finish long before anyone else. My empty plate sits before me like an admonishment. To distract from my evident greed, I tell the entire table about the woman in seventeenth-century dress sitting reading in the little room off the lobby. They stop eating. 'But the flat was built in the thirties,' Gee says calmly.

'Oh, she doesn't come with the flat, she comes with the panelling,' I answer, cocksure. There is an uncomfortable silence round the table. Bit by bit the conversation laps around me and without me again.

Suddenly, as if I have been felled, I can't sit. It's not that I don't want to sit, I can't. My body simply won't stay in an upright position. Ann, ever-vigilant, sees it. I am led away dragging my feet, especially my left foot, which I seem to be unable to lift clear of the ground, into the blissful bed.

I wake and have no idea where I am. I look for the light above the door to my right, and there is none. No sounds either. There is light coming from the other direction. Why can't I hear the nurses talking? The sound of clogs on tiled floors? Ah, yes, this is Gee's home, where

I was before the—where I was before. The hallway's over . . . there . . . I try to sit up. A long business. The hardest bit is leaning on one elbow, half-way up, as the burning neck then has to bear some of my weight. I have to think about how to distribute my weight and where to move my legs. The floor is warm and there are soft woolly rugs on it. I rise shakily to my feet. I hang on to whatever is in reach. I feel very, very old. Not pretend old. Really old. My body feels aged. I fear I will fall. The fear brings a taste of bile into my mouth, which in turn makes me feel sick. For a few seconds I flail perilously mid-air.

Ann appears from her little room next door, heavy sleeper that she is, as she has heard me shuffle my unaccustomed way through the furniture of my pretty bedroom to the lavatory. 'Are you all right?' she whispers, gently pulling stray bits of my fringe in the direction of the shaved bit of my head. I am filled with waves of love and gratitude for her. I touch the stubble growing on my scalp and make to pick off a piece of scab that I can feel has loosened since the last time I tried to have a pick. Firmly she takes my hand away. '*Are* you all right?' I nod my head vigorously to assure her, then wish I hadn't.

In the morning I wake with a pain that is shattering in its intensity. I can't move with it.

It is the mother and father of all the dire headaches I have ever had. I am on fire in the neck muscles that support my head. It makes me catch my breath and gasp. There is a constant grinding background pain, then sharp stabs from a dagger somewhere behind the scar and my right eye.

We have paracetamol to treat it with, which, of course, comes nowhere near even slightly dulling the pain. I wonder if it is the second aneurysm bursting. I wonder if I am going to die. Normally I would dismiss such melodramatic meanderings as the stuff and nonsense that it is, but I did nearly die. What was it—how many weeks ago? I try that thought again. It means nothing and, anyway, thinking hurts. No, the thoughts don't hurt. It's the gaps between them, which I've never noticed before. Trying to shorten those gaps is hard. I can't do it. It is that which hurts.

Ann won't let me have more painkillers than it says on the packet, of course. I count the hours till the next two paracetamol, which also have no effect. The pain doesn't let up. I lie all day in the shuttered grey room with the pale grey muslin curtains twisting gently in the draught from the slightly open window and think, If this is what the future holds then I want none of it.

Bath! A bath. A proper bath. What a delight.

The first in . . . ? 'The first in a month?'

'Five weeks!' says Ann, meaningfully. I remember that we came for three days.

The water thunders into the bathtub. The mirror mists over. I watch, intrigued, as the swirls eat up the cleanness of the glass in waves of smoky clouds that retreat and advance on the cold surface. The steam, damp and moist, creeps into my nostrils along with the heady smell of whatever bath oil Ann has just added to the water. It smells good enough to eat. The foam rises and billows, luxurious and exotic. She tests the water with her elbow. As you do for a baby.

She helps my shaky body off the chair where I have been sitting and I step gingerly into the benevolently warm water. She helps me sit. 'Now, call me if you need help,' she says, retiring with some propriety into her room. I look at the white flaking skin on my thighs, my arms, my legs. I am peeling all over. I pick up the flannel to wash myself and am overcome by such crippling lethargy that it drifts out of my grasp and floats away. I feel myself go with it. My head swims. I hold on to the edge of the bath with hands that have no grip and try to shout, 'Ann, please, please come and get me out.' I have been in the bath for less than a minute and I am weeping and whimpering uncontrollably. I am shocked by myself. No, I'm shocked by this woman who can't sit in a bath for more than a minute.

I have to work in America in seven weeks.

I slump gratefully back into the bed I have only just left.

Bernard comes to sit on my bed. He is debonair and gentlemanly and perfectly proper, but I find his closeness worrying. At least his presence stops me howling. Behind him there is an exotic bunch of flowers in the fireplace from the École Internationale where I collapsed. Something with an extravagant feathery orange tongue is curling out from inside its dark green pod. It seems odd to see such a tropical bloom in the greyness of a Paris winter. The children from the school have sent letters and cards and drawings, all wishing me well. I feel very touched and tearful. Opening them becomes a tiring ordeal. I push them limply into a pile and feel bad. Badder.

Bernard says I am 'vraiment formidable'. I smile weakly. I feel nowhere near *formidable*. He goes on, 'C'est miraculeux. Mais oui. Il faut l'admettre. You look completely . . .' his voice falters as his eyes track up to my head '. . . normal.' This makes me realise that I don't have the scarf-band on: I half-heartedly attempt to pat my fringe over the scar.

'Oh, don't worry about that. As soon as the hair has grown no one will see it.'

'The surgeon shaved my head himself,' I repeat proudly, like a child who has been given

79

special treatment and has learned to recite its thanks well. Bernard smiles. There is a tinge of collusion in it. I say, 'There's a woman reading in the little alcove near the hall.'

'Oh,' says Bernard.

'She's wearing a boned satin dress and a little hat.'

'Ah,' says Bernard knowingly. He smiles again.

'No, no, the hair—it's nothing, nothing at all. You look fine.'

Of course—I'm talking to a Frenchman who imagines, as I am a woman, that this is a prime concern of mine. I have something more pressing. 'I have to work in Denver in . . .' I had worked it out. Which of the numbers was it? '. . . in seven weeks.' I watch carefully for his reaction. I have to work. When I have work my house doesn't seem so empty.

He raises his eyebrows and shrugs in that noncommittal but slightly unhopeful way the French have. He waves something away with his hand, clicks his tongue and changes the subject. 'And you are going home in four or five days, then?'

'Yes, I think that's what Ann said. Ann said I've got to get used to . . . I've got to get used to . . .' An understudy playing my beloved Callas? '. . . to . . . being in the world again first. To . . .' What was the word? Nothing happens in my head while I think. Or, rather, I don't think. There is a void in which nothing

80

occurs until the word pops into my consciousness. 'Acclimatise myself.'

Yes, that was the word. Another lesson well recited too.

'Is that what Ann said?'

'Yes.'

'And she said you are going on the train?'

'Oh, er . . . Yes. I hate flying. The surgeon said I could fly but—'

But Ann thinks it's better on the train?'

'Yes.'

'And you're going to stay at her home?'

'Yes, because I mustn't be alone.' I am pleased I can actually manage to say that word. But I am ashamed to feel tears prickle the back of my throat. 'The surgeon said I mustn't be alone.' Which he did, but it seems as if I have an excuse now, which of course I do.

'And will that be all right?'

'Oh, yes.' I think of Ann's comfortable, well-stocked, well-run home where I've had many a dinner and disagreed, largely good-humouredly, with almost all of her friends. All except those slightly right of Attila the Hun. 'It will be Paradise.'

I open my eyes. My head is clear. The pain has gone. I am filled with an inexplicable joy. My whole being surges with it. I feel blessed, alive, alert, benevolent, miraculously lucky, and just unbelievably happy. I want to wake the whole

81

flat up, the whole of Paris, the world, and say, 'It's all right, I feel all right.'

Carefully we cross the main road to go down to the market in the rue de Passy. Each car that whizzes by takes my head with it. I am not attached to the pavement. Only Ann's arm, with its strong hold on mine, keeps me from floating off in whatever direction takes my attention. There seems to be so much to see. The cold bites through my hat into the scar but there is also something delicious about breathing in such sharpness. Not so the pedestrians. Parisians, never renowned for their politeness, seem out to topple me. People push into me from behind, catch me as they pass, knock me with their elbows or tread on my heels. Every contact is an affront, a burn to the part of me that has been touched. I utter, 'Mais vraiment!' or 'Ça alors!' in the wake of an unseeing pair of eyes, and feel utterly ridiculous, pathetic and livid. I envisage a metal cage all the way round me, a kind of mobile wire-netting tube. That would do it. That would protect me. That is what I want.

There are oysters for sale with fantastic ridges of grey and purply blue in their shells. The lemons beside them are alive in their yellowness. I want to stop and eat the fat tempting lumps of sea-tasting tenderness. To slurp them down one after the other, but Ann

82

urges me on and away. 'People do eat oysters in the street in France,' I want to protest, but I am caught by the rows of fine chocolates in a shop window. I stare till I can taste them dissolving against my palate, and have to swallow all the saliva that has collected in my mouth. I've never really liked chocolates much before. Every shop has a different set of enticements.

There is lacy underwear of such beauty that it makes me gasp with delight. Matching pants and bra in an exquisite shiny satin. I feel ashamed of my old Marks & Spencer's stuff. Even the new old stuff. I want this exquisite smoothness and gossamer filigree against my skin. Only this will do. It is riotously expensive. I am not working. I have no money. Don't think. I feel a rawness in my chest and an ache between my shoulder-blades. My coat feels very heavy. We walk on.

There is a supermarket next to a greengrocer's, which I reel into, clutching Ann now with both hands, my head spinning with the images of row upon row of shining red apples, a patina on them that looks like sheer polish, plump orange apricots, and dates from Tunisia, still on their stalks, redolent with memories of my mother and stepfather's home in North Africa, fat green fingers of courgettes—I seem never to have looked at vegetables and fruit before. I am dizzy with colour and choice. I must buy a tube of the handcream I always get when I come to Paris, the one my mother used. I free myself from the arm and lurch round the aisles, hanging on to the shelves, looking for the familiar pink box. I must have it. I grab it and totter. The bottles and boxes and shelves all threaten to converge. 'Done too much,' Ann mutters at me, and steers me towards the exit where we have to wait and wait. I feel unmitigated hatred for the woman in front of us at the checkout. 'For fuck sake, hurry up,' I say. I am surprised I have spoken.

'Sssssh,' Ann says, with the trace of an indulgent smile.

'They don't understand,' I snap back. I feel I cannot walk another step.

We go next door for a hot chocolate. It's a classy café, recommended to Ann by Gee, that bakes its own bread. The chocolate takes ages coming. I twist and turn to try to catch the eye of the waitress again. I feel cross.

The place is full of BC/BG's (Bonne Classe/ Bon Goût) Parisian Sloanes. I'm glad I'm wearing my fake fur coat. I bought it because it was the kind of thing I thought Callas would wear, except that in those politically incorrect days hers would have been the real thing. I had hoped it would make me feel cosseted when braving the wilds of Bromley and Milton Keynes on tour. Now I'm glad I'm wearing it because it holds its own in here—shades of my real mother (French), always deriding the way

I was dressed by my foster-mother (English). Suddenly I'm unaccountably hot. I can take off my hat, of course. Oh, but I can't. I go to take off my coat and can't. I haven't got enough strength in one arm to stretch it behind me to release the sleeve of the other. I try again and give up. Ann jumps to help. The noise in the café is deafening and I haven't got my hearing-aid in. Don't these people know I've hurt my head? No, I've had an accident. No, that's not right either. But they must be quiet.

The smell of freshly baked bread is overpoweringly yeasty and crusty. Under the lighted counter, safe behind the glass, are glazed fruit tarts, *milles feuilles*, apple puffs, chocolate éclairs, meringues, croissants, brioches, *petits pains*, none of which I can eat because wheat flour makes me ill. I feel very cross indeed. The chocolate finally arrives. I gulp it down and want another immediately. Now. I order it. My order gleans a surprised look from the rather superior waitress and a flicker of discomfort from Ann.

Outside again, the road back stretches away ahead of us, crowds of people milling about blocking the route, crossing the cobbled alleyway, disappearing into shops and popping out again. Coloured shopping-bags bobbing in and out beside grey coats, black coats, blue coats, brown jackets. I feel a swelling fury against each and every one of them.

Instead, I count every step of the way back,

one less, one less, hanging meekly on to Ann's arm, praying I don't trip or fall.

I want to stride into the middle of the main road with its surging traffic and scream at it all to stop. To stop moving. Not just to let us cross. Simply for it not to move. I scowl at every driver as we cross, then beg Ann into walking, or rather dragging me, just a few more yards to where I can see a cash machine in the wall of a building on the corner. I get out my card and panic. Numbers. Numbers have always made me panic. I could bring on an asthma attack at will in an arithmetic lesson when I was seven. She watches me with particular interest. Everything stops for a few seconds, then I recite my pin number. The cash drops out of the machine. I pay her for the mangoes and the avocados, and for the phone calls she's made to England. Ever one to cover a tricky moment, I trot out my National Insurance number and my VAT registration number, just for the hell of it. Number perfect!

Ann grins. 'Not much wrong with you.'

I grin back.

We are going to the Bois du Boulogne in Gee's car. We stop outside an elegant apartment block in one of the wide, gracious, tree-lined avenues common to this uncommon area of the city.

'Do you want to get out?' asks Gee, turning to me in the back seat. I can't think why we've stopped. We're going to the Bois du Boulogne for a walk. 'And *not far,*' Ann had said emphatically, when Gee suggested it earlier. Ann turns round to look at me too. There is a hiatus in the car while my head stops spinning and catches up with the rest of my stationary self. Before I can wonder too long which bit of me to engage in opening the door, Ann has done it. 'Mind your head.' I duck carefully to avoid the car roof and pull myself with some difficulty up on to the verge. I wander shakily towards the rather grand entrance protected by high iron railings.

There is a plaque on the wall that reads, 'Ici décédée le 16 septembre 1977 Maria Callas.' A welter of contradictory feelings invade me. Sadness for her dying here alone, apart from her maid Bruna. Shock to think I nearly died in Paris too. Grinding regret that I never finished playing her when I'd only just begun to know her well and love her so much. A rush of determination to play her again.

I *will.*

I *will.*

I remember the last moments of the play when, having finished her teaching at the Juilliard school in New York, she walks slowly round the stage staring silently into the auditorium, as if it were the last time she would ever stand on a stage. A stage. The place she felt most at home in the world. The glinting gold and red plush tier upon tier of La Scala, the Met, Covent Garden, thousands of lighted candles filling the amphitheatre in Verona. The place where she could be most herself. A stage. I will get back on stage. I will. The force with which I feel this renders me almost incapable of standing. I totter.

I re-enter the real world and sense that Ann and Gee are standing near me, pointing at the first floor and chatting about the building. I feel their closeness as the most acute invasion, and am consumed with ever-increasing waves of rage at both of them.

As I sit in the car I shake. I shake with exhaustion and with anger. I watch my knees jitter up and down. I am powerless to stop them. My left arm twitches. I can't feel my feet. My body doesn't seem connected. There is a throb where my head is. I can feel a tightness in my brain—that I can feel my brain at all is odd—and there's a raw ache in the middle of my chest where something is gnawing away at me. My right hand is numb with holding on to the car door as we jostle and nudge our way through the Paris traffic. Outside there are towering black shapes against the skyline. The wreckage of the worst storm Paris had seen for centuries. Dinosaur-looking dead trees. Huge trunks hurled out of the earth and flung willy-nilly about the place. Long spindly fingers of roots point starkly up into the winter sky. Broken branches are scattered on pathways and flower-beds. All has been left in uproar from the winter storms. It is total devastation. I feel at one with the landscape.

I give my suitcase one last longing look. When I next open it, I think, I will be home. We will be home tomorrow. Well, not home, because I mustn't be alone, the surgeon said so. Home with Ann. What a blessing.

Bernard smiles and says quietly, as he kisses me goodbye, 'And the little lady in the alcove . . . Is she still there?'

I focus sharply on him, to see if he's patronising me. No. His face is sombre. It's a secret we share. I glance over to the small room on the far side of the lobby. 'Yes.'

He smiles wider. 'And what's she doing?'

'Still reading.'

Wheelchair, pavement, taxi. Wheelchair, pavement, train. I feel very important in the wheelchair. A wheelchair is serious. I also feel every bump, every misplaced paving-stone, every bit of unevenness, every gutter, every kerb. My teeth are jarred in synch with the bumps under the thin tyres of the wheels. I am also aware that no one finds a wheelchair worth remarking. We are met with much ado, though, by the railway staff, who take over from one another at given points on the station, like a team in a relay race, while Ann frantically tries to keep up with me and locate the whereabouts of the bags, and my repeating her instructions in French. It is a hectic trundle. Then, like everyone else, we are left to wait and wait and wait for the train.

It moves off, slowly at first. I want to shout with joy at the sheer miracle of it. I think of the days when trains went chusha-puffa, chusha-puffa, and there was a leather strap to pull that let down the window. I think of the unheeded warnings of grit in my eyes as I, daredevil, leaned out further than Margaret at number 81. Co-op corned-beef sandwiches in greaseproof paper. I think of eating them in the biting wind on Felixstowe beach with my foster-mother. She has been dead for fifteen years but, with a pang, I wish I was going home to her. I want her. I want Gran.

I eat everything offered on the menu, and am then overwhelmed by such a need to sleep that Ann generously folds up her coat for a pillow, and after we've worked out that I shall have to sleep on the scar side near the window, rather than sleeping with my head near the aisle and risking it being bashed into by people walking past, she covers me up with my old black fur. I lie down gingerly, wondering if the rocking of the train will dislodge the little sense of balance that I have. I am ashamed I fear so easily for my head.

When I wake we are in England. I look at the rows of semi-detached surburban houses with something resembling love in my throat.

'I was worried the pressure in the tunnel would hurt your head.'

'What tunnel?' I say, and get the laugh I wanted. I am shocked that I have given no thought to what a trial this must have been for her. I just want to get home. Well . . . back.

Waterloo station. Wheelchair, platforms, pavements, taxis, red London buses. Waterloo station. I can't believe it. Grubby, uncharismatic Waterloo station makes me cry. I've never felt at home in London in all the years I've lived here, but these are tears of gratitude for the familiar. My brain must have gone to mush.

We wait and wait for the minicab that the health-insurance people have arranged with Ann. I bubble with impatience. I want to get to Warwickshire. I don't want to think of my home in Putney, just over there . . . Anyway, I'm going to Denver soon and friends will move in. I'm going home with Ann. I mustn't be alone. I've been ill. Am.

The driver seems flustered, apologetic for the delay, and impressed by the wheelchair. It elicits a gesture of extra care and concern from him, until the station attendant folds it up from under me and whisks it away.

We nose our way slowly out of London, my head bobbing up and down more frequently, in time with all the potholes in the London streets. I take to cupping my hands round my jaw to diminish the jarring of my head into my neck. Ann, in best Girl Guide mode, deftly twists her copy of *The Times* into a makeshift neck-brace, covers it with her silky scarf and curls it round my neck. The jarring is almost imperceptible. We laugh. I am grateful, relieved, exhausted, exhilarated, triumphant and utterly spent. There is only a hundred miles to go.

The car is drifting into the hard shoulder. I notice it, as the surface is rougher and my head bobs up and down all the time. I sit up slowly and weakly. Ann is dozing beside me. I look at the driver's face. He seems alert enough. I can't, of course, I think hazily, trust my sense of balance any more. I drift again. Again the unevenness wakes me. I look out of the window on my side, the left side of the car, waiting till my eyes focus with some sort of equilibrium. The Tarmac rushes past under my gaze making me feel queasy. I look away, but catch sight of a white line as the car moves back into the slow lane of the motorway. I look at Ann. She is looking at the driver with a troubled expression on her face. She looks at me. I want to speak to her in French so that he can't understand, but then I remember that she can't either. We say nothing. Moments later the car drifts again. I want to scream and scream. Ann and I catch each other's eye.

We both engage the driver in half-hearted conversation and elicit from him the fact that he has been driving since 6 a.m. It has long gone 6 p.m.

Ann, kindly soul that she is, gives him tea when we arrive and no small warning about his return journey. Meanwhile I wait impatiently for his departure to burst out with, 'A month in Paris in Intensive Care—to be killed in a mini cab outside Banbury?' She explodes with laughter. I manage a quiet snigger.

There are double the number of stairs in the cottage than in the flight I managed some days at the end of the corridor in the hospital. I am beaten, I cannot do it. Ann half pushes, half lifts me up them, while I observe the sound of uncontrollable yelps and sobs that echo round the little timbered bedroom with its pretty floral sheets and lacy pillows. 'Now, now,' says Ann, patting my back.

After my breathing has slowed, I luxuriate in the comfort of the bed, the silence of the countryside, the softness of the carpet. When I wake in the night and Ann comes padding in, she has heard me stir through the half-open door, I tell her, 'It is all so perfect. I feel I have died and gone to heaven.' She smiles.

'Of course she's been to hell and back,' I hear her say, to many of her huge number of friends, who phone her for an update on her last four weeks, though she says five . . .

I can't think about time. It just isn't possible. There was never enough, but now it seems to be bending and looping back on itself. I can no longer understand it. Nor do I want to.

CHAPTER FIVE

Not So Fast

There is a raindrop hanging on the tightly furled bud of a thin black branch just outside the bathroom window. It catches what there is of the light as it is buffeted by a February gust. It lengthens, then retracts. Still it manages to hang on. For a while it is transparent and immobile, till it is caught up once more by the wind.

At some angles I catch the pinks and reds of the rainbow in it. At others it lights up a silvery blue. Now green. Then there is a flash of purple. I watch, entranced. It regains its clearness, like a droplet of pure glass. It quivers. A stronger squall catches it and it is gone. It's not till I remove my hand from where I have been supporting myself on the sink that I feel the stiffness in my back, and realise that I have no idea what I am doing in the bathroom or how long I have been staring at a raindrop.

Spring. And I am alive. What better time to be given another life, I think magnanimously, as I make my way cautiously down the few stairs back into the sanctuary of the bedroom. My toes relish the soft wool pile of the carpet after so long on hospital lino. From the kitchen comes the cheery morningness of Radio 4.

I watch the clouds moving across the window towards a small patch of blue. If it is a good day, there will be a sunset to enjoy later as the bedroom faces west. I eat all the breakfast Ann brings me on the tray. I can't remember the last time someone brought me breakfast in bed on a tray. I feel spoiled and cherished. It is a unique and novel feeling that single mothers don't have, even ex-single mothers like me.

With a paper knife she opens the few get-well cards that have begun to trickle in. I've never opened envelopes like that. It intrigues me. We smile at the cards and ooh and aah at the dedications. Not many people know where I am. She's managed to keep it quiet, so I get maximum peace to heal, she says. She's going out shopping so she's arranged for someone to come in and sit downstairs when I have my afternoon sleep. I'm allowed up for lunch. I have no choice but to go back to bed after it, because my body can't manage to digest the food and keep me upright at the same time. It has taken us several days to discover this, and many half-pushed, half-pulled journeys up the stairs when my legs simply refuse to function without her guidance and encouragement. It shocked me. But my reluctant lackadaisical body has us dissolving in giggles as I remind her of the Monty Python Ministry of Funny Walks.

The sheets feel smooth and silky. I pick up my book. It is my eighth since coming out of Intensive Care. I'm keeping a list. I relish this reading. It makes me feel like the naughty child I was, when I read in bed for hours longer than my foster-mother ever knew. I do keep going over certain paragraphs, though, if the writing is particularly dense, or the sentence structure at all odd. Ann gives me books she thinks aren't taxing. Many I silently deride. Most I can't recall.

We decide what treats she will bring me— easier for me to choose freely, now that I give her money for my keep. I feel better that way. I look forward to her bringing back the Rowntree's fruit gums with only the slightest qualm about putting on weight. But that will go, she assures me, once I start walking again.

I sleep comfortably, deeply, soundly. The Neurontin (anti-epilepsy pills), of which Ann gives me three a day, 300 mg, make me feel drowsy almost as soon as I've swallowed the first with my breakfast. I still haven't quite accepted staying in bed, but I do feel so damn woozy and I know that she's worried I'll fall if I stagger about downstairs. So, like a good girl, I do what she says. Where, after all, would I be without her?

Later in the afternoon I sit by the fire, hemming a skirt that I'm turning up for Ann. I have begged her to let me do something. My suggestion that I do the ironing has been greeted with hoots of derision. But I can't just sit. I never have just sat. I don't know how to do it. I have to get on. I must *do.* So I'm sewing, in fits and starts. I can't put my head down to look where I'm sewing for long and if I hold the skirt up at eye level my arms ache. But at least I'm being of use to someone.

I enjoy the flames licking round the logs, the greyness scurrying by outside as the wind gets up, the sense of warmth and comfort, a sanctuary away from the world. I don't let the world impinge much on my thinking: it's safer that way. Anyway, I've got to get well for my nine-month job in Denver. I've written down somewhere that I'll have two months' rest. Two months? It seems an unbelievable luxury after the maniacally busy overstressed existence that was my life before.

'Of course she's been to hell and back,' I hear her say again, to yet another friend of hers who rings. I wriggle my toes in the woollen warmth of my socks, snuggle deeper into the armchair, guilty for feeling so good about hell.

My son is busy, but he'll be coming again in two weeks' time. He is very affectionate towards Ann and she, in turn, thinks him 'deevine', even though they'd met relatively few times prior to my being ill. Ann and I have only known each other five years, after all. I can only guess at what they went through in the hospital together during all the time I was unconscious. It pleases me that they are close. Without Ann, my son would have had to face it all alone. When he was last here, his father rang from America to speak to me, a comparatively unusual event, but one that has particular significance for me now, as he had kept so regularly in touch with Ann when I was in Intensive Care. He happened to be working in Paris at exactly the same time. Odd.

Downstairs is the biggest bowl of orchids that I have ever seen in my life. They are from him. Well, from his office. It took Ann, a friend of hers and much mutual astonishment to lift it off the ground.

My ex-husband rings when we are at supper. He has rung before, and just spoken to Ann, as

I was asleep or Ann deemed me too tired to hold the phone. Even now I still can't manage it for long. Just talking on the phone takes so much out of me that holding it becomes impossible.

'Thank you for the orchids.' I don't recognise my voice: it sounds quavery and small. It's seven o'clock. That's late for me to be up.

'How are you?'

'Tired. So very tired.' I remember I last said to him I was tired to my bones. What a ridiculously inadequate description, then and now.

'Well, you have just climbed Everest.'

A neat description, I think. It fits my body state exactly. He was always good with words. Words. Work.

'And I'm not working . . . Can't work, worried about money. There's none coming in.'

'You are not to worry about money. Do you hear what I say? You are not to worry about money.'

I am flooded with relief. I entertain the peculiar notion that somehow, now, there is a support system out there that I have not experienced before. Or in the eighteen years since the divorce. A sense of family pulling together in a crisis. I have a sense, too, that somehow, if that's the case, it has all been worth it.

99

I feel strangely content, and very near tears as contentment is a beast that's strange to me. Ann recognises the warning signs and at a signal from her, she and my son lever my floppy body out of the chair, hitch me up the stairs, undress me for bed—an act I find strangely poignant as it doesn't seem *that* long ago, to my exhausted mind, that *I* was undressing *him*—and then we all sit back rather self-consciously and survey the scene. My son's departure is always a dangerously significant time, so while he extricates himself to work a bit on his laptop before bed, Ann begins the nightly treat of telling me the story of What Really Happened. We have gone over what I don't recall time and time again. I look forward to it. It's like a bedtime story. Like a child I know where all the questions come.

'So when I fell . . . ?'

'You didn't fall, you had a fit.'

'A fit? But the kids at the school—'

'The kids weren't frightened—we'd made a circle round you.'

'But when I was sick in the gym . . . ?'

'No, we had lifted you into the school library by then.'

'So I was sick in the library?'

'Well, you were out cold first —'

'I've never fainted in my life.'

'—for a good half-hour.'

'Half an hour?' I repeat, in my child-like voice. Where did I go when I wasn't there? I wonder.

'Dr Vinikoff said not to worry about the bits you can't remember. There will be bits you can't remember.'

'When he sat on my bed in the ambulance, and told me I might die?'

'That was in Lariboisière, after you'd been scanned in the other hospital.'

'What other hospital?'

'The hospital the ambulance took you to first.'

'*Then* I went to Lariboisière?'

'Lariboisière was on duty that day for emergencies.'

'They have the best brain surgeons in the world.' Again I am the good child, repeating her well-learned lessons. 'The ambulance men were lovely, weren't they?'

'Do you remember them asking if there was epilepsy in your family?'

'No.'

'Oh, you had a good long conversation with them in French.'

'Oh.'

Pause.

'I wouldn't know about the epilepsy in the family bit anyway, not being conversant even with my father's name.'

Giggles.

'Why do we never hear about people with

aneurysms?'

'Because—'

'Because most of them are dead. Most of them die.'

Silence.

'I'm very lucky, aren't I?'

Ann nods and smiles, pleased.

Again I am flooded with gratitude, taken over by it.

'You were quoting reams of Shakespeare.'

This is an old routine too.

'Not reams! I quoted one line . . . I remember it—when they tied me into my bed. It's not even from a part I've played, very odd. I remember saying, "Bear-like they have tied me to the stake: I cannot fly."' I think, I'll never live it down, quoting Shakespeare in Intensive Care.

Ostensibly time passes me by. I don't know what the days of the week are. Or where I am in the week, I only know I measure time backwards, by the number of days since leaving hospital. The few notes I have managed to scrawl on odd bits of paper, hardly a diary, bear testament to that: '6 weeks and 6 days since op', '2 weeks "home" minus 2 days'. At the front of the back of my mind are Denver, and getting through the check-up trip to Paris just before. I daren't count the weeks to Denver. I keep trying to luxuriate in a sense of space that stretches out before me, timeless. It's a novel idea. Space and Time. I don't seem ever to have had either. Now that I have them, what exactly they are seems to elude me.

The tree outside the bathroom window remains stubbornly black and bare. Beyond, the relentless greyness mocks me: if it threatens rain I'm not allowed out for our little walk. For a few days now I've been crawling along on Ann's arm to the end of the lane. When I turn I can still see her front gate. The long walks of my past, scrambling up hills, walking for hours across windblown fields, whatever the weather, line up in my mind to mock me too. I don't feel like laughing back.

I cannot force my body to go one step further than it will. An odd experience for me. I have spent years galvanising it into doing what I wanted and needed it to do. Now I don't even seem to have the galvanising wherewithal. Often I count the steps back, each one more arduous than the last. Sometimes my left foot drags just slightly on the road, which confirms Ann's modest assessment of the distance to be correct. Damn her. Damn.

There are startling green buds on the blackthorn along the lane that I latch on to with avid eyes, but I'm not allowed to stop, even though I'm wrapped up like an Eskimo, a scarf round my head under my hat to protect the jaw where they took out the piece of bone

103

to get into my skull. Sometimes it clicks alarmingly out of place, but I've learned how to click it back again. I won't allow myself to wonder what would happen if this occurred on stage. When I do, I think it could be very funny.

I am not allowed to drive. In case I have a fit. Ann says a year. The local GP doesn't seem to know. Ann drove me there, then came and sat in the doctor's room with me. I felt six years old again. I am to have physiotherapy at the local hospital. They think it a good idea. I am signed off sick for the first time in thirty-five years of working life. I get fifty pounds a week. I give Ann sixty. It's only right. We're both independent working women with our own homes to run. Except we're not, not now. We used to be. She's retired and I can't work, and friends are going to live in my home in London when I'm in Denver. Another friend is waiting to be installed in the cottage I rent just up the road. I'm living in Ann's home. I repeat and repeat this to remind me what my life is. What is my life? No work, no car, no home. No big deal, I think. I've been here once before when I was ill. Not having those things doesn't change who I am in essence, I think. I can handle it. I think. As long as I don't think too much.

As long as I can walk. Walk a little on my

own. And be brave enough to shut the bedroom door when I try to meditate first thing in the morning. Like I used to do. In my other life.

I put up the ironing board when Ann is out, determined to do the whole load, to be of use. I stand, driving myself on to do one more piece, and then another, the way I'm used to challenging myself. I complete less than half the basket and have to sit down as I can no longer deny I feel woozy. I collapse into a nearby chair, trembling slightly, which gives way to shaking with exhaustion and body-racking sobs.

It's only the ironing. But it seems redolent of so much else I can't do. Who am I now, if I can't do what I used to do?

The local cottage hospital becomes a place of sanctuary and succour. The physiotherapist's strong hands ease the stiffness and pain in my neck and work the flabby muscles in my back. A month in Intensive Care has not only made me shed the layers of skin that are normally brushed off by clothes and showers and just the friction of living, but caused all the unused muscles to hang on the bones. That's why, when I'm tired, I can't sit up or stand up without help. She works the base of my spine where she says the blood from the bleed in my head will have collected, until it is dispersed back into the system. I picture my spine clogged with blood like flesh left on a fishbone. She is very delicate when she goes anywhere near my head. Instinctively I flinch, but there's really no need. What a drama queen I am. Was. Am.

It is the first time I have been touched with care and gentleness for weeks. As she works deep into the bones and joints I feel a sort of awful ecstasy. A pleasurable pain. Tears trickle down my face into the hole in the bench where my face is. I can see them darken the floor beneath in spots. Her kindness and attentiveness make me weep, but she's seen it all before. In her professional mode she hands me a Kleenex, says, 'Have a good cry,' and gives me some very gentle exercises to do on my own each morning. I leave grateful and exultant. I have found a friend who understands my body's needs and pains, and at last I think I can begin to help myself.

I writhe around on the floor in my bedroom dutifully each morning, appalled at the waywardness of my limbs. Without her discreet and pivotal help, my arms and legs are in disarray. If I wasn't so frustrated, cross, hot and bothered, and just plain pissed off with myself, I could laugh. I must look like an inept octopus.

I demand, on my son's next visit, that we all

three go to get the cottage ready for the friend who will live there when I'm working in Denver. The kitchen has been redecorated after central heating was installed and things, I insist, must be returned to their proper place. The resistance this suggestion meets is only to be expected but is no less wearing for that. Ann says it's not necessary, that the friend won't know where things ought to be. 'But I do,' I maintain. My son, recognising when my mind is made up, sways the vote in my favour. We go. I haven't been to the cottage since the Christmas before collapse. BC, I think wryly.

It is only three miles up the road from Ann's home, so any jarring to my neck and head in the car is minimal. She drives carefully, with her attention on the bumps in the road, of which there are many—she's had practice in getting me to the doctor's and the hospital. Seeing this landscape, which I know and love so well—the hills I walk often, palely sketched in the distant mist—sets my emotions on a helter-skelter. Everything so familiar looks so different, so startlingly new. I hear myself talk and talk and talk. Each word depletes my already dangerously low energy level. I seem unable to stop.

Inside the cottage I am determined not to cry. After all, they'll be proved right if I do. It's mostly the idea of being 'home' and the silly little trinkets and things I have been given over the years, which I love, that threaten to set me off. The glass jug from the church fête that cost 50p, the white pottery doves on a mobile that hangs from a beam, photos of loved friends, who don't know where I am, that I haven't seen or spoken to since . . . AC (After Collapse), I suppose, only that sounds rude.

My son, having moved all the furniture back into place, knowing I will be content to potter, warns Ann off with a look that I catch. I am at last happily alone in my beloved bolthole to dust and reacquaint myself with this bit of my life and jiggle things about till they're where I like them to be.

I lose track of time but they don't. I must have been standing for over an hour. They had told me to sit down but I forgot, I was so absorbed. I forgot I am ill. On the way out of the back door with my son behind me, my legs give way. They simply are not there. I am in space. The speed with which he is at my side, grabbing my elbow, hauling me up from falling, and the accompanying look of grey, strained terror on his face, is, I suspect, a vivid, momentary encapsulation of what I couldn't see during all the time I was unconscious.

The next morning I can't stop the tears. I wake up feeling wretched before I find out that he's gone. Sensible fellow. I whine with pain. He is the person I most want to be with in the world. He is the only family I've got. I miss him more than I can tolerate. It is like a gaping, gnawing raw wound in my chest. I cry like a six-year-old. I am inconsolable. Ann says, 'He has to get on with his own life.' I want to slap her hard. This renews the tears. I feel pathetic, overwhelmed and desolate. I am also full of self-loathing because most of these tears, which I can't stop, seem to be for me. But I don't know why. Ann pats my back and there-there's me, but I won't be there-there'd. I want to be with my son. I cry till my head throbs. Then I have to stop. I try to sleep by reading yet more. I can't not read. That would mean just lying there doing nothing.

Later, Lise rings from London to give me an update on the house and how things are there. I shouldn't have taken the call, of course. Ann usually filters who I talk to, but we both misjudged this one. I am overwhelmed by my life at this end: the idea of London, mail, bills and the garden overgrown is all too much and I find myself shouting at Lise down the phone. Not just talking loudly, shouting. I don't do that with Lise, ever. I pay her to look after things in London when I'm not there. She works for me, and either side of that work we don't have that kind of friendship. A yelling, telling it like it is friendship. There's too much I can't or couldn't say. Not now though. I shout louder and louder. What I'm shouting nevertheless seems to me to be reasonable and truthful. I am spiralling with injustice, fury, and distress. Snot and tears run down my face, I sob and gasp for breath as I try to fit in the words between sobs. I am haywire. I argue, I criticise and find fault. I say the unsayable, till she shouts back. I stop. I am so shocked I stop. Lise doesn't do that either, ever. I cry some more and say I'm sorry. I don't know why I'm saying this. I think, I'm the one who's ill. I am racked with an unhappiness that I didn't know I was harbouring. It pulls me up short. I don't know where I am. I want to be anywhere but here, but there's nowhere else to be. It's awful of me not to be grateful. I am grateful, I am, I think, but the conviction is growing that mostly I am awful. I certainly am sick. Sick of myself.

The local vicar calls. Ann had asked if I wanted to take communion, as he does the full travelling service. At first I thought, Yes, then I realised in time, that with just him and me, he would hear all the words I won't and can't bring myself to say because I don't believe them. So he came and just sat on the bed and we prayed together, or at least he did, because I couldn't hear what he was saying, and didn't have the courage to tell him so. Although I don't know the man at all well, I am comforted by his presence and his genuineness, and I feel safe in the hands of a professional health carer, so I voice one of my greatest concerns: 'How will I ever pay back this gift?'

He surprises me utterly by saying, 'Perhaps you've already paid it.'

For a while this consoles me. Then I remember that, in spite of what Dr Vinikoff said, it is all my fault. As my foster-mother, whose voice I seem to be aware of frequently these days, would say, 'Now look what you've brought on yourself.'

The physiotherapist tells me I'm doing well. I shrug it off, impatient with myself for not doing more.

'I can't even sit up without help.'

'Well, it's early days yet,' she says.

Early days, I think poisonously, it's been weeks and weeks. Why aren't I well yet? My body's never had this much time off, I think grudgingly.

'It's hard for people like you who are used to being busy all the time.'

'I'm not a workaholic,' I retort sharply. 'I take time off—I walk.' I think of Ann commandeering the pathetic two-hundred-yard strolls. 'Well, I *used* to walk,' I snarl . . . 'I sit by my cottage fire . . . Well, I sit by the fire in Ann's home.'

I think of Ann sitting patiently in the waiting room.

'I mustn't be alone.'

'It must be very frustrating.'

Suddenly at this moment of unexpected sympathy my body jumps, a jolt like the sense of falling as sleep begins, except this jolt has started in my body not my head. I give way to waves of what can only be called grief. I am astonished at how quickly it envelops me. I try to get my head above the Plimsoll line. I snuffle out an indistinct, 'What was that?'

'That's all right, just let go. It's the massage that makes you give in to it.'

She hugs me, there is kindness and understanding in the hug. It's not a professional gesture and the tears increase—is there no end to these damn tears? I am so weary of them and they bring such exhaustion in their wake. I worry about the noise I must be making and how it must be disturbing others, if there are any, on the other side of the flimsy curtain that doesn't quite reach the floor.

'Why the hell did I jump like that? It happens sometimes when I'm resting on my— the bed in the afternoon. It's not a falling-asleep fall . . .' I snuffle out between sobs and phlegm-filled snorts into a handkerchief.

'Your body might well have a memory of when you fell.'

I remember my first encounter with a memory held in the body. How I couldn't shake off the arthritis with which I had played Piaf at night for weeks in the West End. I would go to pick up something at home and see my hands diminish into the twisted claws I had learned to use for the latter half of Piaf's life. Not deeply attractive but I wasn't going anywhere or doing anything else. Till filming *Cleopatra* during the day at one point for BBC Television. I used to joke about it and say my Cleopatra was the only Serpent of old Nile with arthritis. I don't feel like joking now. The memory of Piaf and Cleopatra makes me cry even more.

'I am so fed up with myself.'

'Are you overdoing it?'

'I'm only knitting and reading,' I answer bad-temperedly.

'Well, that's a lot.'

'It's nothing at all,' I snap. I don't mean to snap. I like this woman and her helping, healing hands, but it's out before I knew it was going to be a snap.

'It must be so hard for you.'

I think, Oh, please, don't show me any more sympathy or I'll be off again, and the tears don't bring relief.

'Hard because you've lost all your independence.'

Prescient on her part, as only days before I'd written as a note to myself, still not able to write a proper diary, 'Before I was lonely but independent, now I'm not lonely but am totally dependent.' It seemed a ridiculously neat and uncomfortable equation.

'Yes, it's hard because I'm a bolshie, difficult, rebellious sod,' I interrupt. The irony of this description being so way off the mark, given my present state, is not lost on me.

'And hard for Ann too,' she says.

I writhe inside with discomfort at this. Everyone can see how good and kind Ann has been, is being, is. Landed in the thick of it in Paris with with three days' worth of clothes, no French and a would-be corpse for five weeks . . . She says it was five weeks, I think it was only four. Why does time do this looping and doubling back on itself when I try to sort it out? I must work the timespan out. My head whirls in spite of the gentle pressure at the base of my neck coaxing and easing the rigid congestion away.

'It's hard for all carers.'

Something resembling rage begins to bubble inside me at the injustice of this. I think I manage a half-swallowed 'What?'

'It's very hard for all carers to let go.'

CHAPTER SIX

Oh Yes I Do.
Oh No You Don't.
Oh Yes I Do.

The radio is shouting downstairs. There is an undertow of people talking too. The indistinctness feels like a long, low rumble of drumsticks to the skull. Every word from the radio feels like a pickaxe prising open my soft brain with a piercing acuteness. I get out of bed slowly, trying to keep my awareness attached to my body and away from the noise. Every movement jars my neck and head. I push away *The Times* with its urgent headlines in disgust. The brusque movement makes me wince. There are piles of cards and letters on the tray. None with a Los Angeles postmark or a flash of ex-husband's cash. No money yet. I sit on the edge of the bed and watch the floor recede and advance. Gently I raise my head and focus on the open bedroom door. I lever myself into an upright position. Slowly and quietly I shut the bedroom door leaning on the door handle for support. I reach the little bench eventually, sit and try to meditate. I have started my day by trying to meditate for about twelve years but I haven't been able to sit up without help till now. I have looked forward to this, to getting back to my old routine, back to my old way of life.

I can't shift my awareness from each of the aches and pains. It seems that every area of my body is screaming for attention. When I close my eyes, flashes of darkness and light go off and on and off and on and off and on. I want to shout too. It's unnerving and unsettling, this change from light to dark over which I have no control. What chance have I over my thoughts if these visual fireworks unbalance me so? I struggle to catch my breath.

The bedroom door opens. I feel myself

115

gasp. It is a violation of my privacy beyond anything I have ever experienced. I can't make the joke about matron doing her rounds. Or even the one about visits by the bedroom police.

I am awash with rage. I am in a turmoil of fury. I say nothing. How can I? If it wasn't for Ann where would I be? I hear the echo of my foster-mother asking, as she did often during my childhood, 'And if it weren't for *me* where'd you be? In a home.'

The door closes. I am flooded with adrenaline, which makes my heart bang behind my ribs.

Breakfast on the tray has appeared, as do lunch and supper every day. Every day I eat it all up and feel grateful. Today I feel venomous. Helpless, dependent and venomous. And fat. I can't get my dark green trousers done up. I shall have to move the zip. If only I can keep my damn head bent over the sewing for long enough. I'm quite good at sewing, but today even the idea of it seems an insurmountable problem. But walk I will.

I have to sit on the bed to put my socks on, which takes an infuriating age. I used to pride myself on my yoga-like balancing on one leg at a time. Now I puff and pant and have to pull each foot towards me with both hands, wincing at the burning in my neck as I move my head.

'And where do you think you're going?'

I am stopped at the bottom of the stairs, so rotund with layers of clothes, I can hardly turn to address the voice. 'Out for a walk.'

'But we go for our walk just before lunch.'

I have seen this. The moment I've been dreading. 'I'm going now. I'm going to the village shop.'

'But that's miles further than we've—you've walked so far.'

'It's on the flat. There are no hills. It's all on the flat. It's only a couple of miles.'

'A couple of miles!' Ann is so incredulous that I am momentarily daunted. *Is* it a mad idea? 'I've got to go. I've got to go a bit further every day. That's how I tick. I have to challenge myself . . .' I can hear my voice getting dangerously strident in pitch, there is the stinging of tears in the back of my throat, and under all the layers of scarf and waistcoat and vest and cardigan I am raving with heat and determination.

'I'll come with you if you just wait till I've—'

'I want to go now. I'm going now.' Shakily I make my way out the door. I despise myself for not having the courage to say, 'I want to go alone.'

Outside, the lashing of the wind against my face feels good. It makes me gasp, catch my breath, and I need to steady myself on a hedge, which gives with my weight. Out here, in the world, I feel I have the ballast of a feather. The flat empty fields stretch away on either side of the road in sharp ridges of brownness. Where the plough blades have left a smooth slice of earth there is a tinge of purple and silver that catches the little light there is in the grey. A winter landscape usually lowers my spirits. Today it enchants me. Green spears of daffodils, their buds still hidden, pierce the grass of the verges. The blackthorn has stretched a few more brave pleated fans of vivid green along its black, spindly warp and woof. Above, there is so much sky. I breathe deeply, look up cautiously and feel a sense of the hugeness of the space into which I launch a heartfelt thank-you. I am alone for the first time in months. Apart from the mind, all is quiet.

The shop has been forewarned by phone of my arrival and are insistent that they drive me back. I am equally insistent that I walk. It takes a lot of energy to be insistent and polite. More energy than I fear I have. I can feel a hole where my guts should be and a red-hot brand between my shoulders. I sit and drink a welcome cup of tea and try not to want to keel over into the armchair, curl up there and stay. For ever.

I walk back. I am triumphant and more frail than I ever thought it possible to be. It takes days to recover from this walk.

During which time the man I am about to work for in Denver, Peter Hall, phones. It is late, six-thirty, sevenish. My supper is wreaking its usual havoc, taking all the blood from my brain to digest it, rendering me almost comatose and, physically, almost immobile. It is my first experience of talking to a 'boss'. I can't get out of my head how I must sound to him. I monitor the conversation. Am I slurring my words, as I do sometimes now when in the grip of this crippling fatigue? Am I making sense? Have I got any words back to front as I sometimes do now too? I engage my professional self and do a performance of a woman who has not a care in the world and whose one object in life is to work in Denver for nine months. Only the latter half of this is true, of course. Apparently I perform it well, or he's too practised to allow his misgivings to show. I can't, however, dismiss the paranoia about my behaviour being scrutinised, and not just by me.

I feel exhilarated by the prospect of going away for nine months. A new group of people to work with, America—whose energy I've always found attractive—a major new theatre project written by John Barton, to whom I owe and love much. A new life. What could be better? A new life when I have a new life?

I mull this over as I knit. The red trail of scarf grows longer and longer.

Try as I might I can't quite picture myself standing by my bed in London with an open suitcase and piles of packing. Two, three, four open suitcases? How do you pack for nine months? I have trouble remembering what's up the road in the cottage that I might need and what's here with me at Ann's, let alone what's in London. Denver is six thousand feet above sea level: how will that affect my brain— my eyes, even? They dry out easily since the cataract operations. Supposing . . . The thoughts topple and jumble into each other, chatter and shout, demanding attention I don't have. My head spins. Downstairs the radio talks. Downstairs Ann and some friends are talking. I want to run away from the noise in my head. I want to run away. My whole body twitches and jerks, a huge staccato jump. What is it, this mammoth jolt? It's like a huge electric shock. It frightens me and shuts me up.

I shout and scream, and shout some more. Ann and her friend Bea are on the bed, both stroking my one free hand. I am on the phone. I am livid. My son, at the other end, is saying that going to Denver is out of the question. 'Ann knows it, Bea knows it, and I know it,' he says. I look at both the faces, questioning. Ann and Bea nod sagely and sadly. I feel paranoid and conspired against. This knowledge that they have all shared without my knowing separates me from the self I thought I knew, and the self they seem to know. It makes me

120

feel isolated. Frightened. Worst of all, trapped. Trapped and tamed by this new and unknown person.

I can't talk to Peter Hall in this state. This state takes its toll and its time.

'So.' I swallow. This is hard—it's harder talking than I ever thought possible. 'I could push myself, like I've always done—like all actors do—but it just wouldn't be fair on my son . . . and Ann . . . and . . . everything they've gone through. It would make a nonsense of . . . everything they've had to *watch* me go through . . . that I didn't know about . . . It would make a nonsense of . . . all the pain if . . . by working too soon . . . I got ill again.'

And that, more or less, was that. It took me days and days, lots of scraps of paper and many Kleenex to boil down what I had to say to Peter Hall. To reduce it to its bare minimum. To keep going over the points in my head so I didn't wander off the subject, come the day when talking to him on the phone could no longer be delayed. To be on my guard against him offering generously to start rehearsals later and to give me more time, both of which he did. On my guard most of all against my saying in response to this, 'Oh, yes, fine, all right, then, I'll come.' And then my life would be back. I'd be back to pushing myself through fear, like all actors do, back to blocking the aches and pains with painkillers,

121

back to the old life. I would know who I was again. No actor in their right mind would turn down nine months of work. But I don't know what life I have now, or who I am, or what mind I am in.

'Sure-fire way of giving up smoking? Have a cerebral haemorrhage!' It gets a big laugh from everyone in Gee's sitting room. Mostly from dear Bernard who's been very solicitous since our arrival back in Paris for check-up brain tests and a visit to the valiant Vinikoff. I've come armed with a large book of pictures of the most beautiful places in England as a present for Dr Vinikoff. It had seemed a good idea in the shop, exquisite pictures and not much text as he doesn't speak English. It was an impulse-buy in a quiet bookshop in Burford, where I'd also craved some new clothes—like an addict, I had to have them— and, having tried on shoes, trousers and a shirt, had left myself with precious little energy for book-browsing or standing up unsupported. Here, in Paris, it seems ridiculously inadequate as a present for saving my life but, then, I suppose anything would.

After we'd got over the jokes about 'We've come for three days but we might stay four weeks!' ('Five,' said Ann, from the other end of the corridor, and I make a mental note that I really must sort out this timescale some time soon), Bernard astonishes me by asking quietly, as we make our way from the lobby to the salon of Gee's apartment, 'Feeling trapped?' I make no reply.

I continue heatedly, frightened of losing the thread of this later conversation, 'People who've never smoked have no idea how hard it is to give up, do they, Bernard?'

'Sssh,' says Ann, motioning me to be quiet.

I want to slap her.

I have to take some ghastly-tasting medicine, which Gee has kindly collected from the hospital, just in case the MRI scans aren't clear, and they have to inject me with a liquid for a CAT scan. I bluster and fume and argue the toss about the ridiculousness of a possible connection between the CAT liquid and my wheat allergy, to which this medicine is apparently the antidote. Gee and Ann watch me bluster and fume from a safe distance, silently. I swallow the stuff ungraciously and bad-temperedly and feel even more like the six-year-old I seem to have become. The silence confirms it. I wish I could hide in the hole I have been digging for myself.

We are kept waiting for two hours for the IRM scan which is the French way round for MRI. I've paid for it—at the hospital cashier's desk, no queue, no fuss—before we descend into the bowels of the hospital where the scanning machines are. Four hundred and fifty francs, it cost. That's forty-five pounds. In England, privately, it costs four hundred and fifty pounds. How long the NHS wait is doesn't bear thinking about. Again, I thank my guardian angels for allowing me to cross the Channel before the great axe fell. The difference in price is not surprising, but this wait is. French hospitals run like clockwork. There would be stampedes and riots if they didn't.

There are only two other people waiting, two elderly ladies, perhaps in their eighties, obviously sisters. I wonder what they make of the three of us. Gee with her lovat-green swagger coat and brown Stetson. Ann with her dark-framed glasses, tie-at-the-neck blouse and navy blue brass-buttoned coat, and me with my crazy-patterned cardigan and blue cloche pulled down to my eyebrows to hide my ever-burgeoning spiky white hair round the scar. My head is whizzing. There are no windows in the room, which feels close and claustrophobic. I find Ann and Gee's nearness oppressive. I have no energy left to rise above it, and that is my own fault. Yesterday I walked too far. I knew it, but I just had to do it. I thought, As long as I go through the motions of what I used to be able to do, then I am who I used to be. I think.

I take off my shoes like all well-brought-up girls, then curl up on the comfortable, cushioned bench along the wall like a *clochard*. I close my twitching eyes firmly so that I can't see any disapproving looks. Secretly I relish my vagrant-like behaviour.

When I'm finally admitted to the scanner, the young technician apologises politely and profusely for the wait, but they had a *cas d'urgence*. I can't imagine this *politesse* taking place among the scuffed walls, seedy corridors and moulded plastic chairs of British hospitals. Lariboisière is, after all, a state hospital, not a carpeted private medical hotel.

'That's OK,' I tell him—his politeness is catching. 'I was an emergency case too.'

He smiles deferentially.

'Dr Vinikoff saved my life.'

He smiles proudly, we share a bond.

He gives me the earplugs, which I insert, and helps me into the small tunnel of the scanner. The noise, which resembles the thumping, whirring and grating of several pneumatic drills just behind my ears, could never be comforting, but its familiarity holds no fears for me: it's almost like an old friend.

We had walked round the Île de la Cité on the day off between the tests and the results. Then we walked round the Île de la Cité again because I lost my bearings and didn't know

125

where I was. I had hoped to go to Montmartre with Ann that night, but Gee had arranged for some of her friends to come round to dinner. 'And she was so kind to me all the time you were in hospital I can't really go against what she wants,' Ann had said. I argued with her about not losing her right to have a differing opinion just because someone had been kind, that it was sentimental to think like that, and nonsense to hand over one's power, but I knew I wasn't really talking to Ann at all.

Gee's actress friend, whom I'd met the night before I collapsed, didn't turn up after all for dinner that night, so I was alone among people who had regular incomes, stocks and shares, and who knew nothing of the lottery of jobs and income that is an actor's life. I felt very separate.

'Do you never lose an argument?' enquires Gee, rather tersely, the next day as we are having a drink in a café where we are killing time before the hospital visit to see Dr Vinikoff and get the results of the tests—Gee is coming too, to translate for Ann and explain to me. I know she doesn't mean this remark as a compliment, even though it's dressed up quite disarmingly. I seem to see through people now.

'Gee, I'm not arguing,' I say testily. 'It's about engaging, it's about having a proper discussion instead of just social chit-chat.' I am generalising and making a mighty sideswipe, that I know, but actually I don't really know what this is all about at all. I feel surges of fear about the tests, and great, suffocating waves of frustration and irritation about everything else. Something is very wrong.

London had flashed past, a blur of intolerable noise, strobing lights and swarms of people, which had, even from the comfort and protection of Ann's car and her little mews flat, overpowered and undermined me. I simply couldn't handle being in the city. The city where I had, have, my home. Now, from the safe distance of Paris, London has been reduced in my mind to a sharp, potent memory of my flinching and clutching a banister, and then Ann, to avoid being toppled over by a crowd of schoolchildren at the National Gallery as they had surged up the stairs towards me. We were seeing 'Seeing Salvation'. I saw red. I spent most of the time hating the people who were in front of me at any picture or sculpture. Not just a mild irritation, a naked loathing. They were in my way, they got too near, they talked too loudly, and I didn't feel at all uplifted. I looked at most of the stuff quite dispassionately, I felt no connection with the Divine in whichever form it was presented. Most of my time and the energy I didn't have were taken up in feeling malicious about the entire human race. Then the train journey, more traffic, more people, noise outside, noise inside, perpetual movement, perpetual stimulus that beat my spinning, exhausted brain with blow after blow.

Here Parisians, in their determination to get where they are going, indifferent to all around them, unnerve me even more. Their confidence sets me reeling and wanting to lash out at everything. I have to keep talking, pursuing my train of thought, although I have no idea where it's leading. I just can't seem to let go. Again I am back in the two-of-them, Ann v Gee, and the one-of-me-situation, and I don't like it—I don't like it at all. There's not much I do like nowadays, I think, then feel guilty that I'm not feeling grateful for this life I nearly didn't have, and feel even worse for thinking, It's not much of a life.

Dr Vinikoff takes the book shyly, and puts it discreetly to one side with an almost indiscernible smile. There are MRI scans hanging on a white screen. He points to various bits of my brain. I gather that the second aneurysm is negligible at three millimetres. No need to operate till eleven millimetres—if ever. Three millimetres seems to me an awful lot of space to be taken up by something that shouldn't be there, but the mere idea of going through what I've just been through again holds such terror that I obliterate it instantly from my mind.

'And America?' he asks.

'Oh, I'm not going,' I reply, as easily as declining sugar in my tea, and feel again the unmistakable smugness of a child who has got a lesson right. Oh, I am a good girl. This is instantly followed by feeling hot with shame at remembering the flare-up that preceded my reluctant decision. I am convinced everyone in the room can see and feel this too. I am ashamed of my duplicity. I decide, there and then, that it is imperative for me to do and speak only the truth.

On the way out we pass a young man in a wheelchair, whose mouth is open, filled with a lolling salivating tongue, and whose legs are evidently useless. It seems a significant sight, which adds to my shame. When my face has stopped burning, I feel humbled. It is a lesson that is driven home hard.

At the end of the Paris trip I get to administer my anti-epilepsy pills myself. Ann shows me how. All the pills for one day go in one of her little boxes. That's what they used to do for patients when she was a nurse. Then it's easy for me to see what's gone. Do I see? I see more than I admit.

There are dozens more get-well cards and flowers awaiting our return. No money from America in the mail, but a surprise bonus nevertheless: I have an income insurance, which I had forgotten about and which will pay

129

out a small amount each week after thirteen weeks of illness. Some God-given accountant must have bullied me into it during my salad days of working on TV. It won't cover my overheads but it will bring in a little something every week—not a comforting regularity with which most actors are familiar, even successful ones.

I take up the red scarf with a feeling that borders on pleasure.

Just to balance out the sense of ease with which I envisage the weeks ahead of me; a God-given chance to rest for once in my adult life—seeing them at last as weeks of space, not weeks of unemployment—my VAT papers arrive. I look at the pile of receipts and papers—shoved anyhow in what used to be Jamie's office—all of which have been untouched and disordered for almost three months, realise that the numbers and columns of figures mean absolutely nothing to my befuddled, overtired brain, and collapse in shuddering yelps of despair at being beaten yet again by things that 'normal' people cope with perfectly well.

Ann has cleared a space in what used to be his office for me to work in. I don't like it. It's cold and bare, not really part of the cottage. I pretended I was pleased to have it. So much for truth. It is, I suppose, somewhere to escape to. But it has no door. I watch my tears darken the tooled leather top of the large desk.

130

Guiltily, I rub them into the gold-patterned edges of the leather in case Ann should see, but, defiantly, I snap on the second bar of the electric fire. Easy: No.

One Saturday evening, I suggest we go to Ann's village church the following day. She seems disinclined. The idea goes no further. Consequently I sleep late into the next morning. I wake to thin April sunlight. As I come down the stairs—I now make my own breakfast—Ann is ready for church.

I take it into my head that, once she's gone, I will walk back to my own cottage. It's only three miles, after all, and I have been building up to it, walking alone now almost every day. It is the only thing I can do alone. I have an overpowering desire to see faces I know and places I love in my own village. I plan to buy some cheese and an apple and the Sunday papers from the village shop and sit in one of my favourite spots on a hillside and pass the day just being. I don't plan to visit my cottage, as that would mean talking to the friend who is there, and I know that I am in dire need of a day of silence.

The road is busy, it being one of the first fine weekends of the year, and each car that whizzes past me threatens my precarious balance. The sun feels strong and good on my face, and I feel my spirit expand in the silences between the hissing of the tyres close by me on the Tarmac and the peace that folds in after they have passed. The road seems to have more bends in it than I remember. There are daffodils out in sunny spots among the roadside bushes, which would be hidden from view in a car. I take them as a personal gift. My elation grows. Then I feel dizzy. Then I feel frightened about falling down on the road. Then I am chastened that I now scare so easily about the slightest damn twinge. I give myself a good talking-to and plod on. When I arrive the village shop is closed. I spin with indecision. My whole day is changed. What will I do now? What can I do? I take myself off for an apple juice in the pub to rethink my day. I have to sit outside as the noise and laughter inside are more than my jangled nerves can bear, and I am frightened someone I know will see me and want to talk. It dawns on me that I don't have the strength for a single word. I don't know how long I sit clutching the diminishing lukewarm liquid in the smeared glass.

I walk slowly up the hill towards my cottage, knowing I can't go much further, and realise from the empty driveway that, thankfully, no one is in. I call out to a neighbour ahead of me, who greets me with such a welcoming genuine pleasure that a few moments later I find myself in her kitchen crying in response to her sympathetic questions with the all-too-familiar tiredness but a new, acute sense of relief. She cradles my head against her and strokes it with a gentleness I didn't know she had. I chatter and stammer and blurt out all the bottled-up distress I didn't know I had until, having fed me cheese and apples, she tucks me up in a blanket in a comfy armchair outside in the sun and, by some miracle, feeling very blessed, I sleep.

More mail, more heaps of cards, but no money.

Hello! magazine wants to interview me about the collapse. We plan all sorts of elaborate set-ups, mostly with Ann in the forelock-tugging yokel or serving-wench role. I know she's secretly pleased at the prospect of having her exquisitely decorated cottage photographed. I see it as a chance to earn a little. Underneath the feeling ghastly I am tickled very pale pink. I didn't think they thought I was famous enough. Once I suggest a fee they don't. But it sets me and my agent thinking. I decide I *will* do the interview apparently requested a good while back by the *Daily Telegraph* just to prove I am alive, if not exactly kicking, after all.

This proves to be arduous beyond belief, not least because it means travelling across London on my own, in a cab I can ill afford— the little pension doesn't kick in until 13 weeks of illness—and pretending to the journalist that I am well and not at all nervous, which she, of course, sees through and describes rightly as the performance that it is. I talk stream-of-consciousness and have no overall view of what I'm saying, and have made no choices about what I do and don't discuss. It's all spontaneous and instantaneous, until I'm halted by her asking, 'Why don't you ask your ex-husband for some money?' I manage to field this with a 'Perhaps you'd like to write to him on my behalf?' but the closeness of the brush with danger makes my hands shake. It isn't hard for me to hope that my ex-husband will send me some money, as I asked for nothing when we divorced. But to have a journalist so near a subject so precious is very frightening.

It is also the first time I have seen my much-loved agent and her two assistants since I collapsed. The reunion is as uplifting as it is emotional. This young woman had to handle all the professional flotsam and jetsam from my collapse—cancelled performances, producer, press, and company manager constantly on the phone, as well as the many friends enquiring where the hell I was. Rumours, too, apparently from one source, which I learned of much later, that the brain haemorrhage was a cover for a nervous breakdown. (I plan to accost this person with an offer of a prolonged feel of the scar.) With an agency representing largely young actors my agent has had no practice for this kind of responsibility and, from what I can gather from my son who was much impressed, handled the crisis with great aplomb and total truth.

After the journalist has left the office and there are hugs all round and many smiles, I thank my agent for the great job she has done. Her open face with its candid gaze says, 'I just told them you were expected to make a full recovery.'

I am expected to make a full recovery.

It's a phrase that echoes round my head for days after my visit to the hellhole that was London. The cab I choose to blow away more precious money on for the return journey seems to hit every pothole in every well-pitted street. I have never been aware before of the startling lack of suspension in London cabs. My head aches. I fumble for painkillers in my bag and swallow them with just a dim shadow of something that resembles guilt. I have been here before.

I am expected to make a full recovery

Am I? Haven't I?

Was I ever not?

After London life becomes more disjointed than ever. I feel dissatisfied and dependent. I am irked by all I cannot do. Can't drive. Can't work. Can't cook. Can't go out. Up till now I haven't cared. Now I do. I don't feel safe in this sanctuary any more. Outstaying my welcome flickers regularly through my mind. My discomfort grows in proportion to my sense of guilt. I don't want to be here any more. I can't lose my awareness of the real world lurking just beyond the door.

Two friends visit, bringing the world even nearer. I can smell the outside on their clothes. It makes me nervous. Ann and I do our double act again. I go through the story twice more. Ann adds the bits that have become silently acknowledged between us as her contributions. I try to limit descriptions of the pain to one of these friends, who has been in a wheelchair for twenty-five years. Perhaps not surprisingly, she also doesn't pick up on my sense of feeling trapped. Ann's kindness receives another paean of praise. I dig myself another pit of guilt. The second friend, Caitlin, who happens to be the one who is going to move into my house in London with her husband, Richard, and who *does* pick up on my dilemma—it's her job after all, she's a Jungian therapist—ends her visit with an emphatic 'Never, ever, underestimate the seriousness of what you've been through.' This strikes me as odd, because I still don't quite know what it is I am through. I feel uncomfortably at the beginning of something.

A few days later I receive several pages of fax from her about the 'hero's journey through many vicissitudes'. I feel flattered, but I don't feel at all heroic. I feel grumpy, ill and full of ugly, pent-up rage. Something bad is in the air.

The washing-machine overflows, and I try to give Ann a hand clearing it up. Not easy to keep bending down to floor level. She snaps at me. I snap back and taunt her with her oft-repeated lesson to me of it being as gracious to receive . . . It becomes increasingly difficult to deny my sense of it all being wrong. It has grown until it clamours for attention. If our friendship is to survive I must go. I know I have outstayed my welcome. I must go, but where?

Days later I find myself storming at Ann as she stands cooking my evening meal. She screams at me. 'Do you make *all* your friends scream at you?' I am shocked. She hardly ever raises her voice. Something in me gloats at this and something else doesn't recognise the bit that is gloating.

When the newspaper interview comes out I find it gratifyingly honest and reasonably well reported—no mean feat with today's journalists ever on the lookout for the easy character kill with which to draw attention to themselves. Some days later the journalist forwards a letter from a GP in Marlborough, who's taken exception to two points in the article. She goes to great pains to explain that an aneurysm *isn't* a ruptured artery, but a swelling on the artery wall with a consequent thinning of the artery, which increases the *risk* of rupture and haemorrhage. Then, having described the aneurysm as congenital—which, according to the GP, is correct—I had proceeded to say that as my mother did not have one I must have inherited the weakness from my father (whoever he was). This elicits a line of capitals: 'CONGENITAL IS NOT THE SAME AS INHERITED'. I burn with shame that I have got it wrong. I worry, as the GP does, that parents will think they have passed something on to their child—that it is their fault. But I *know* it is my fault. And now I have to bear that I may have given it to my son. 'Congenital means existing from birth, e.g. an extra finger. Hereditary is something passed on from one's forebears.' I stare at the letter for ages. Try as I might, I cannot see the difference. I apologise by return of post to the journalist and explain that 'It is beyond me. I cannot understand it. But then I *have* had brain surgery.' I hope this will make her laugh. It doesn't make me laugh, not in the slightest.

Later I have even less to laugh about. Ann and my son, together and individually, complain hotly to me about the newspaper article and my behaviour. I am aghast. Neither of them liked being mentioned. I don't understand it. I have told the truth as I promised myself I would. She *did* borrow my underwear. She *was* a nurse. He *is* my son.

What's the big deal? What have I done wrong? I have simply told the truth. I am stunned, too, that they are not filled with praise for my having managed such a stressful thing at all. They, of all people, know how frail I've been. Am. Especially as the London experience drives me into bed for a considerable part of each day for a long while after. I try, unsuccessfully, to rest and lick my wounds. I toss and turn, feel very raw in my chest and jangled in my head. I smoulder over the injustice of their judgements, feel paranoid about the unity of their reactions and deeply hate them both.

I have a brainwave. I will go to America. I have dear friends there whom I love, who I know love me. Brilliant idea. America will do me good. I'll be ready to go back to work when I come back from America. I always feel energised and positive after a visit to America. One phone call to my astonished friends in St Louis establishes that America it is.

I write to the friend in the cottage—I don't trust the constant residue of tiredness from the London trip to allow me to manage the phone—to say that I would like to move back in when I return from America in early June. This gives her plenty of time, two months in fact, to make other arrangements. She moves out two days after receiving my letter. I am stunned. I have no choice but to move back in immediately as I can't afford to pay Ann for my keep and the rent on the cottage. I have to speak to this friend on the phone the day I receive her letter and what I say, which seems to me perfectly reasonable and, what's more, utterly truthful, makes her scream and howl. I am horrified. I don't know why. I slam down the phone as if stung, while she is still screaming. I shake. I don't know what to do. If I were still smoking I could light a cigarette. I am terrified at this change to my plans. Change floors me utterly. I can't handle change. The idea of having to pack up and move out of Ann's seems a mountainous task. I want to be alone, but how will I manage having to be alone in the cottage? Well, at least if I fall, I think there are people who pass by who would see me. That is no comfort at all.

I am terrified of being alone—not just in case I fall. I am terrified of this person I seem to have become. What is it about me now that makes people react like this? What am I doing?

My cottage homecoming would have been joyous if I hadn't felt so grim. Patricia and Shirley, friends, had filled the fridge with food and cleaned the place from top to bottom. Friends who have cleaning ladies of their own. This nicety is lost on me. I just want to get all the stuff I have accumulated at Ann's unpacked and stacked away and then to bed. My own bed at last. When I do I cannot sleep. My body is in turmoil. It won't let me alone, however much deep breathing I try to do. I am tormented, what by I do not know. I've got my independence back after all.

The next morning it hurts to move but washing must be done, especially as I have the luxury now of doing it myself. I used to see it as a chore. After loading the machine—it hurts to bend—I stand up too quickly for my tired brain and crack my head against the low beam in the kitchen. I gasp. The blow is right along the scar. I gasp again and wait to fall. I don't. But I hear the wailing yelps of a hurt child.

The village shop-owner greets me with delighted smiles and hugs. Pleasant as it is, I am overwhelmed by her show of joy. I feel I hardly know her. Then I realise I have used up all the strength I have just getting there. Outside the shop a kindly soul says, 'Are you better now?'

Exasperated by this first encounter with the appalling ignorance about brain injuries and daunted by the return walk of some five hundred yards, I snap back, 'It's not flu I've had, you know.' Another social triumph.

Sleep continues to elude me. Or my body does its jump and jolts me into consciousness again. Exhausted as I am, the moment my head sinks into the pillow, my brain reruns all the scenes of the collapse that I can recall. I

141

wasn't frightened when they happened, but I am now. I can't shake off the terror of wondering how I'll manage to get through the day if I don't sleep. It doesn't matter how many times I tell myself it doesn't matter that I don't sleep: I'm not working, I don't have eight performances to get through, I can sleep during the day. But I don't want to go to bed in daylight. Only ill people go to bed by day. But I do want some respite from the ugly jangling of my thoughts. Shut up, for God's sake, woman. Shut up! I shout at my head.

I'm washing my hair under the kitchen taps —a relatively rare and tentative experience still as the scar seems to draw and pull at itself if I lower my head—when I hear the church bells start up their ringing. Thinking I might find some comfort in the peace of the mellow Cotswold-stone chancel, and some guidance in the words of the communion service—relevant bits have a way of jumping off the page—I run upstairs to dry my hair, gulp down my breakfast, then rush across the village green down the little alleyway into the blessed peace of the Norman church, as I have done many times before. There are about five worshippers assembled, most of whom turn round and smile a greeting. I feel welcome and glad I came. The vicar enters and the service begins. The words of the Eucharist sound distant. Then the run makes itself felt. I burn and become uncomfortably hot. Sweat starts to

142

trickle down the sides of my face and neck. I dab at it ineffectually with a screwed-up paper handkerchief that I find in a pocket. I then turn icily cold and know that I am going to pass out. I know what it feels like now. My hands start to shake and my legs turn to liquid. The terror is quite palpable, especially as the woman I am standing next to, Judy, turns to look at me with some concern. She takes hold of my elbow and the kindness in the gesture makes my knees sag and my eyes fill. From somewhere behind me another kindly hand, René's, proffers a paper cup of water. I am shaking too much to hold it myself, but gulp it down gratefully like a child and sit feebly through the rest of the service hearing nothing. I have frightened myself again and, worse, all those around me. They now know I am still not well. I know I must get help.

I decline the local GP's choice of a neuro-surgeon and choose instead a consultant in London I had liked when he treated a stage injury. He has been kind enough to agree to take on my case and will validate my not driving and fill in the forms for the DVLA. He thinks, as Ann does too, that a year must elapse before driving again after a brain injury. I am outraged. A whole year. How will I manage? My car is my freedom and my independence. It turns out that it is only six

143

months—if I haven't had a fit. So far, touch wood, I haven't. My useless car sits like a rebuke outside the house in London, exactly where I left it on 9 January, but I don't care. My not being allowed to drive means nothing in the face of feeling so incapable. There are days when, having pottered round the kitchen, I can't walk even to the village shop. I ask my son to move the car to the cottage and get it off the road to save me money. The thought that legally I will be able to negotiate London traffic just weeks after my return from St Louis appals me.

David, an exceptionally bright and honest friend of mine, more than makes up for his not being allowed to visit me in hospital in Paris, by driving me from the cottage with my suitcase for America. On our way to London I watch his face to see if it betrays recognition of the difference I feel. He seems to relate to me as he always does, I think. Or if not he's too damn clever to show it. I lose track of what I'm watching for and feel self-conscious about staring at him. In no time at all he is gone. I am at home alone in London. I wait for my passport. While I wait I think. I try not to. Not to think of what would happen if I fell. If I fell I would stay on the floor until the cleaning lady or Lise, who does the mail, comes in and finds me. It is a worrying thought. One night I

144

feel so sick and dizzy, I make up a bed with towels on the bathroom floor, rather than risk falling down the stairs in an effort to get to the loo quickly and not spray vomit everywhere. Vomit means burst aneurysm. I am not sick, however, and get fed up trying to get the sleep I so badly need on the hard bathroom floor. I give myself another good talking-to for being a drama queen and head back to the relative comfort of my bed, where sleep, as ever, eludes me.

I wait and wait for my passport to come back with its work permit from the American embassy. The friends in America have suggested I teach one masterclass, and the university has sent me the air ticket on this understanding. Usually I teach for a month. As each day goes by the level of my anxiety and discomfort increases. The departure day draws near, and I still have no passport. I double up on the sleeping pills and still read most of the night. I potter restlessly about the house during the day, getting it ready over and over again for the friends, Caitlin and Richard, who will live there occasionally while I'm away as they would if I had gone to Denver.

When the passport eventually arrives, I hug it to me in relief as if it were my reprieve from prison. All will be fine in Am-mer-ri-ca.

Now, only twenty-four days after I should have gone to Denver, I am going to Missouri. I can't quite get my mind to understand this bizarre equation as I wander into rooms on a mission and, once there, have no recollection of what that mission is. When I do remember, I often find the chore already done. I stare at the clean sheets already in the spare-room cupboard as if they have been whisked there by unseen hands. My conviction grows that I am not alone in the house. I try to deride it as fanciful nonsense, but my new sense of perception won't allow me to dismiss it. The house certainly feels different, but that's perhaps because Caitlin and Richard have stayed here once already. She has said that, lovely as the house is, she finds a negative atmosphere here somewhere. I wish she hadn't said it. It doesn't help my insomnia one jot.

Her husband has rearranged my little garden. Window-boxes have been upturned and emptied, beloved plant pots moved to different spots. I spend most of the afternoon I arrive home dragging or lifting all the pots back to their original places. I drip sweat, although the day is cool, and puff and pant, but I am possessed by the thought that things must be as they were. 'Negative influence?' I fume. The only damn negative influence is Richard interfering with my lovesome spot.

I feel the after-effects of this physical exertion for days. I still can't meditate, even in the room in which I've sat for years. And I am too busy getting through each day, too involved with managing the real world, to stop and pray. I still offer the occasional word of thanks into the air in rare moments of physical ease, but what the fleeting gratitude is aimed at I have no idea. At a time when it would seem that, as a recipient of such grace, I would have an acute sense of the Divine, I have never felt more distanced from it. Most of the time I feel too ill to pray.

As the plane takes off I pray. I usually do. But this time I pray because I feel things moving in my head. The contents of my head tighten and loosen and shift. It's subtle but nonetheless alarming. The man sitting next to me doesn't look like the kind who would welcome confidences about brain haemorrhages, so I have to keep it to myself. That's an unusual occurrence these days. To date I've told the woman at the checkout in Sainsbury's, the window-cleaner, Malik, the kind Pakistani who runs the corner shop, and the minicab driver who brought me to the airport. In fact, I can't think of anyone I happen to have met that I haven't told. And that's just the strangers. I can't seem to talk of anything else. I made a crack at the security scanner asking them to allow me to bypass it. It was one of the first things Dr Vinikoff told me was perfectly safe, but I'm not risking it. 'It's not that I'm worried about setting off the alarm,' I said, 'I just don't want to die in the departure lounge of Gatwick

147

airport.' That got a few smiles. I don't feel like smiling now. I am frightened. Not just by the plane. I am frightened of myself and the time bomb that has become my brain.

CHAPTER SEVEN

Head Help

My body lands some eight hours later and is hugged and greeted by my dear loving friends, Henry and Patty, but it is several days and blessed sleep-filled nights before my stunned head deigns to join it.

During the six weeks that I hide in the haven of my friends' home in St Louis, I make myself walk several blocks most days. Past gardens brimming with shoulder-high azaleas in riotous shades of pink, magnolia blossoms the size of dinner plates; all this fringed by a sea of dogwood trees, their white flowers lilting in dense waves that stretch far into the distance of each sun-dappled street. Not hard to find benevolence on such days. The gentle wind billows out my T-shirt. I feel like a little boat. But there are days, too, at this time of the year, of such intense humidity, when the sky is iron grey and oppressively close, when walkers avoid the pavements and stay in the comfort of their air-conditioned cars till they are level with the shop front then make a leap for it, when my constant frailty matches the grind of the relentless weather and I stay in the safety of my air-cooled room. Its windows on the third floor give out on to the branches of a tall, leafy tree, and I gain comfort from its all-enveloping greenness. It's like being in a tree-house. I sit and stare out into the leaves, for minutes on end, startling the occasional bird that perches there; the flutter of its departing wings echoes in my chest. I scratch and scratch and scratch my head. There is nothing on the scalp. It must be the brain beginning to heal and irritate like any scar.

The masterclass passes in a dizzying mist. My body, which reminds me constantly of its presence, is still aching from the flight and my brain is dazed by being under scrutiny in front of a group of people. I have no gumption. I can't seem to galvanise myself. Then my hands shake uncontrollably as the first surge of adrenaline hits my lower back. I have no idea of what I'm saying. Or how helpful or relevant it is. I switch to professional automatic pilot. I say what I've said before, which to any discerning eye may not be applicable to these particular students' needs. I wonder if they can see how strange I feel. Afterwards, the Performing Arts department is full of warmth and generosity in their response, which I measure in proportion to their knowing that I have been seriously ill. It is so overwhelming to

149

see so many bright, loving faces brimming with welcome and relief that I am yet again, shamingly, near tears. I turn over the expressions of relief again and again. Does my escaping death hold something for them too? There is something in that, but it eludes me. Later, I worry that my hands still shake, but I welcome the shred of comfort in knowing that at least my professional response was still there to activate. I remembered what I teach— what I used to teach. I say, when we get home that night, 'A few more brain cells then, not gone under the surgeon's fingernails.' Obligingly they laugh. I love these people.

Once on the scent of the memory issue, I need to know some more. After all, no memory = no job. So, when a timely request comes, I master my initial reluctance and say yes: I *will* devise a charity recital to raise funds for the first Shakespeare festival in the city. It gives me something other than my pesky health to think about. But the jet-lag and the tension of the masterclass leave what's left of my bewildered brain unable to make decisions about which bit of text to choose or where it goes. It's the kind of decision I've never had to really think about till now. That in itself concerns me. I spend days on end pondering the *Complete Works*, distracted into reading bits of plays I've never read before, enjoying being absorbed in it, then coming to and staring in alarm at the blank sheet of paper in the typewriter. There's something wrong but I can't quite capture what it is.

In performance, which takes place in the comfort of the house, I decide to keep the file of speeches nearby in case the words desert me, although I have made an agreement with myself only to resort to it in dire need. I read the bits I planned to read and dare myself to do the rest without the comfort of the text. My voice, now free of cigarette smoke, is fluid, flexible and clear. It is also unrecognisable and unmanageable. This adds to the strangeness of the experience. My whole body judders quite perceptibly through the entire forty-five minutes, which distracts me occasionally from the words, but I get through the evening with only the slightest damage to Lady Macbeth and an almost negligible tuck in Cleopatra. I feel triumphant, stay up too late, drink too much and talk a lot. Then follow several days of living in the void. Physically my body feels beaten with an iron bar. Every joint aches. No position I rest in feels comfortable. My brain, which, disconcertingly, I can still feel, can't follow even the trashiest of the thirty-six TV channels. I resort to watching Judi Dench and Geoffrey Palmer, at least it's what I know. What I used to know. But it reminds me of England, and my dread of going back there grows.

I have to make a detour to Montréal on the way back to England for the Globe. A big firm's bash. They want some Shakespeare acted (me) and some academic info, (Professor Andrew Gurr.) With no further work to occupy me, apart from the speech to write for Montréal, I start almost looking forward to the mail arriving from England to give a shape and purpose to my day. Normally this is an intrusive chore. I go with Henry, my host, and chair of the Performing Arts department, to see a prize-winning play written by an Indian student at the university, and am completely disoriented by it as it is about second-generation Indians born in America so, of course, there is no reference in it to colonialism. Henry and I talk about it afterwards with several others from the department. My assessments don't seem that different to the others', although I reap a few surprised looks at what I'm beginning to recognise as my bluntness. I feel in touch with my capacity to analyse and dissect a piece of theatre writing: that ability is still in place. The idea grows that it's easier to locate my professional self than the personal one and, disconcertingly in tune with this observation, a phone call from Paul Jesson in England, suggesting I do a poetry recital with him and Norman Rodway in Stratford in the summer, gives me a tad more professional comfort. When the idea is mooted that I do my charity

Shakespeare show once more in St Louis before I leave, I am nudged into believing that some direction seems to be confirmed.

Well, at least the speechwriting will keep me out of the shops. There are few shops locally, so a natural limit has been imposed on the extravagant amounts I can throw away on clothes I don't need but have been buying at a regular and alarming rate. I seem to be obsessed with decking out this new body in new apparel. Quaint, the American use of this old word. I stroke velvets longingly, run my fingers over the rough threads in raw silk, let lace slip through my palms, the sensitivity that is still in my left hand allowing me to feel textures in a way I never have before. I'm aware of the gazes I elicit from the shop assistant. I'm aware, too, that the disturbance in my gut, the nebulous fear, is also more acute. I seem to be frightened of everything and nothing. I buy myself a miniature plastic brain which winds up and walks across the table on flat, black plastic feet. I play with it incessantly and show it to everyone. I also buy a postcard that advertises a 50s film, in lurid black and red, 'the brain that wouldn't die.' I photocopy it and write copious letters to friends on it.

I have not heard from Ann or from my son. I do, however, hear from Caitlin, who's in my house in London. She has a problem. Richard, her husband, finds Lise's visits to collect my mail intrusive, Lise herself aggravating and my cleaning lady incompetent. I have a problem. Richard. He then adds insults to my injury as I am taken to task for not having put drainage in my window-boxes and for having put a tablecloth on my own kitchen table. He can't bear it. It reminds him of his childhood. I explode with disbelief. It is monstrous. It is mad. I fume and rage some more. I walk my tree room. I wish I could laugh. I can't. Tablecloths and terracotta! I boil with wrath. I can't contain it. It takes me over. The real me knows this is petty, but I don't know where the real me is. Caitlin's words, spoken on our little stroll in Warwickshire, echo coolly in my overheated mind: 'Never, ever, underestimate the seriousness of what you've been through.' I am no longer sure who's mad.

Each of my days is accompanied by a lump of habitual anxiety in my chest. Nights are a torment. Deep breathing can't shift it. It can't slow my jumbled thoughts either. My mind drifts this way and that, grasped by the worries that lurk just below its surface. Most attempts to calm it end in tears, tears of fury, despair or desperation. Sometimes storms rage outside too. The humidity of the nascent summer collides with the coolness of the departing spring. I jump. I wake. Thinking that my body has done one of its involuntary leaps, I reach for the current book, then cringe at the crashing crack over my head. The sky is split. I

154

watch in fear. The flashes light up the huge satellite dish of a local TV station on a nearby roof. There is an eerie moonscape quality in the weird silhouettes and blueness both outside and in. The crashes lunge closer to the roof. More cracks overhead. I flinch, then hold my breath while angry rumblings retreat across the sky. The night ticks by. I feel the time pass. I switch on the light and look at the clock. I think, I have had more time off now than since my son was born, twenty-six years ago. I must be feeling better. I am not.

There is a limit to how many tears I want to drip on my dear friends so, one rather eye-swollen morning, when Patty and I happen to meet up in her kitchen, I acquiesce to her very American and highly appropriate suggestion that I put myself into therapy. The chance to talk about all this can only help, and putting a finite limit on the time that I do talk about it will be better for us all, especially if I'm going to go back to work in England soon after my return. Maybe September, I think, yes, September, that's always a good time to start work. Four months more of rest. I gasp mentally at the idea of four months being such an easily acceptable slice of time. Not long ago four weeks off would have seemed a lifetime of unfillable space. So, I'll start again in four months. Well, not start—continue. Pick up where I left off.

Beloved Callas . . . I shy away from the

surge of tiredness and the feeling of defeat that this name triggers in my chest. It frightens me. Callas frightens me. I frighten me.

So, therapy it is. Patty knows someone, of course. Sod the money it will cost, I think. I'll sell the house in London. I need help. I make the idea of therapy (only mad people need it) more palatable to myself by calling it post-trauma shock therapy. On one of my endless sorties to the shops—well, the alternative is to walk in the opposite direction and sit in the cathedral, but the Divine and I are badly out of tune, I don't know why—I find myself buying a scrapbook with large, mesmerising coloured pages, and lots of coloured sticky paper to make pictures from. I last did this at primary school.

I am cutting out a pair of black spectacles and some white underwear when Patty shouts up the stairs, 'Your ex is on TV.'

I zap the channels to find the face I know too well, which has so dominated many years of my life, hurl a 'Send me some money, you mean sod,' at the TV screen, scratch my scar, an almost hourly occurrence nowadays, and carry on, between scratches and getting glue tangled in my sprouting hair, cutting and pasting in my Former Trauma book.

I put all the dissidents behind a white wicker fence and let the coloured cut-outs do what I wish I could dish up in words.

Mulling over the past, hearing an occasional

childlike chortle, I get brainwaves for the future. I write to a priest I know about the so-called negative forces in my house, to a friend I haven't seen for ages to enlist her experience and help in flat-hunting and selling the house in London, run lighthearted to the postbox, then curl up on the bed and sleep a sleep of vivid dreams for most of the afternoon.

The Night Sea Journey. Little ship of death. Brown prow, indenting the green page. Death of old life. A gift. A miracle. A chance to change. Rebirth. No. New life. Change. Chance. Honour the new life. The unpeeling of a layer. Friendships unravelling. Stop. Black page. A wake-up call. Red balloon of blood. A warning. Honour the gift. Away from the known here. White magnolia blossoms. Here with the unknown. Dogwood trees. Cut more leaves. Cut. 'Now the eyes of my eyes are opened and the ears of my ears really hear.' Like it to be true. Unlikely to be true. Stop. Really? No. No intimacy, no audience. Odd idea. Alone. In reality. Truth. Really alone. Really truthful. They are not there for you. No money. No love. What safety-net? There are lots of strong feelings here. We have to stop now. Cut. Live in the pit. Live with the pain. Extra sensitivity great strength. Usually. What's usual? Now zero tolerance. Rudi Giuliani. Don't haul yourself up by your bootstraps like you usually do. We have to stop now. Stop. Every day is different. Who is this?

Cut. How can I? Stop. Why does she? 'The unexamined life is not worth living.' Cut out white underwear. White. Black. Off. On. Light. Dark. Shadow. So much shadow. Who? Here. How do I? Get some control back into your life. Why did she? What did you get from it? Fancy implying some ulterior motive! That wasn't what I meant at all. 'No greater treason to do the right thing for the wrong reason.' Repression, depression. Control freak. Don't get sad get mad. Brain hurts. Used to be a joke. Can't laugh. Sad. Mad. Joy. Sun. Leaves. Trees. Bumper sticker: 'De Nial is not a river in Egypt.' Laugh out loud. In the street. People pass the mad girl. Mad girl smiles at flowers. Scissors cut white lazy daisies. Scissors clip scar. Time. Six years old. Tears splash. Thirty years adult woman. Decisions based on wisdom. Step back. Misjudge space. Not back. Falter. Down. Drained. The gift of time. Stop. Pivotal point. Step back. Don't rush it. Stay in the pain. It transcends the son. Archetypal loss. A break, from life. Break. Use the oars. Watch out for the shoreline. The river is too wide to see. Silence. Need quiet. Quakers. Only silence. Rapids. Hold the sides. Hold on for dear life. Dear life. Wasn't. Now? Gift. Drained. Give thanks. Need? No deal. Spooked? Distant. Needs boundaries. Distance.

Need to put some distance to all this bull. The issue is your recovery. Not their understanding of

158

it . . . Abandonment. You have been through abandonment before. You are sitting in it right now. Don't be intimidated by the pain. It will pass. All will pass. (Talmud.) 'That deep torture may be called a hell, Where more is felt than one hath power to tell.' Heart hurt. Break. Sharper than a serpent's tooth. Heartbreak. Perhaps now with him out of the way there will be room for a man in my life.

'Getting smart fast,' he says.
  Not smart enough.
  'Or fast enough,' I say.

CHAPTER EIGHT

American Brain

When I surface enough to luxuriate in the strengthening sun, be pulled by the captivating English sheepdog through the carpets of wild violets in the local park and try to relish the empty days that stretch ahead of me, I realise with some dismay that I feel bad most of the time. My time here is nearly over and I feel bad. Not bad, ill.

'But it's *four months* since I've been ill,' I protest to Patty one day, as we're heading off to do the school run in the jeep. I love these times we have together. She drives languorously and well. She tells me of the time before American cars had air-conditioning, when her father would bundle them all into the back of his open truck, and drive in the cool of the evening so they could catch any passing breeze before they went to bed. We're accompanied by a local radio station that plays songs we know. 'Tamla Motown!' we yelp in delight. No longer are we women over fifty. We giggle as we sing along: 'Walk Away Renée'—the Beach Boys. 'I Get Around.' 'Perhaps some people would say it's *only* been four months,' she says soberly, as we run out of words we know.

Crazy, I think. What does she know? I feel ashamed. Who is this dismissive truculent girl I carry with me all the time now? I love Patty and I know she loves me. That's why I'm here. What does she know? A little voice replies, 'What do *you* know?'

Holocaust Remembrance Day. I go with Henry to the synagogue. Very moving service. The four survivors of concentration camps who live in the city are helped up to the Bema by granddaughters or grandsons to light a candle each. I look around, swamped [as I am] once more. Tears splash down many faces. How do you mourn six million lives? There aren't enough words. There isn't enough grief. My burden feels negligible.

160

I need to go and see a doctor, not a mind doctor, a brain one. After all, a therapist deals with the quirks of the mind. Injury to the brain and what that specific injury causes is a brain surgeon's thing. Patty knows one, of course. He's a friend. I've met his lovely, lively Latin wife several times. She's a drama MA student at the university. She sent me flowers on Mother's Day; another odd occurrence. How did she know?

I compile a list of burning questions for a brain surgeon and don't get the chance to volley one.

He's gentle and big and quietly spoken. I trust him instantly. He's like Dr Vinikoff. Calm and in control. I guess you have to be if you're carving up people's brains. I look at his hands. My brain would feel safe in those, I think. It doesn't feel safe in mine.

'Where was your injury?'

I point vaguely to the right side of my head. He smiles. 'No, I mean which artery.'

I realise, with some concern, that I don't know. Or if I did I have forgotten. Can't forget. Mustn't forget.

'Have you had double vision? No, that's good. Have you lost your sense of smell? No? OK. You have just had the most invasive

161

surgery there is. You have chemical meningitis, which is an inflammation of the lining of the brain—'

He sees my face drop at the M-word.

'Not *viral* meningitis. Chemical, probably caused from all the drugs they poured into your brain to keep you alive while they were operating. You will also be suffering from irritation because of all the blood collected in your spine and neck.'

'Umm-er . . .'

'Yes, cerebral irritation will make you feel irritable. Are you on any anti-epilepsy drugs?'

'Neurontin.'

'Well, you can stay on Neurontin for the rest of your life,' my face drops some more, 'or you can try to diminish the dose and see what happens. If you have a fit it won't last more than one, three, five minutes and when it's over you'll be OK.'

He says it so quietly, and in such a matter-of-fact way, that I think, Yes, I will be OK. The stone floor of the cottage flashes in front of my eyes. I dismiss it. A fit in a rehearsal room? All right for Chekhov. Not so hot for Oscar Wilde.

'I'd keep the second one scanned every six months. I operate at six millimetres.'

I make a hurried mental note to ask the neuro-surgeon in London to make another appointment for another scan for me. 'Dr Vinikoff operates at eleven.' I feel pleased that at last I'm using the vernacular.

162

'Did he suggest an EEG?'

'Umm, er—yes.' I know I've heard this arrangement of letters, but they swirl around my head with MRI, CAT, ECT. No, that's not right. That's the barbaric treatment for depression.

'The French are very keen on EEG. It won't tell you anything.'

I wish I'd brought a tape-recorder. I'm having trouble keeping up with my notes.

'You're exercising?'

'Walking.' The idea of going to a gym is ridiculous, with my head, my back, my neck . . .

'How much?'

'Half an hour a day.' Bury the lie. Feel pleased. Flush hot.

'Do more.' All my life I've been told I do too much. Try too hard. 'You'll know what you can do.'

But I don't. I am completely at sea.

'I have to have medicals for a film.'

'If a film company really wants you they'll get you.' He smiles at me again, reassuringly. I don't feel at all certain about my working on film. It was pretty tentative BC. Suddenly all the years of my working life dart in front of me and seem to perch on high, white-fringed waves, then swoop and dip perilously in the choppy waters. Everything seems at risk.

'You'll know what you can do.'

Later, in his smooth silent car which matches him perfectly, I tell him about the turbulence with friends.

'Oh, we call that the ripple effect,' he says, almost smiling, almost dismissive. Wish I felt it was so minor. 'Friendships unravelling' is what the therapist calls it. I think I swept misgivings under the carpet before. Now there is no carpet. And no time for friendships built on sand.

'Everyone who's closely connected to a brain patient goes through a major upheaval in their relationship with that patient in some way after surgery.' I wonder wryly how many more of my friendships are lined up to go down the lavatory. 'I'll get my office to send you some of the support-group information.'

A support group, I think, what a brilliant idea. Find out if others are as obsessed by it as I am. Just in time I remember to ask him about my jaw. It's ridiculous, of course, because he can't really inspect it as he's driving. It seems he doesn't need to.

'They took a piece out to get at your brain.' This is a statement.

'It clicks.' Not a big problem for a bank manager or a landscape gardener, but could prove problematic on a large vowel on a moan in a Greek tragedy, if I ever get to work in the theatre again, I think tragically.

'It'll settle. It's soft tissue. Soft tissue moves. All in good time.'

164

Time, ah, yes.

And now the sixty-four-thousand-dollar question as we draw up outside my haven at Patty and Henry's home: 'How long will it take for me to get better?'

'It can take six months,' he says, calmly reversing the car into a space. Another eight weeks of feeling ghastly. I feel depleted by the mere idea of it. 'You'll know when you are ready to work again.'

I'm working again in Montréal next week. I almost say it out loud, ever one to come back with a snappy rejoinder. This is largely to attempt to drown the crashing reverberation in my chest set up by his last words: 'Or it can take up to two years.'

I row heatedly with my son by phone; separate from Ann by very calm letter as coolly as the six weeks' silence allows; cry, unproductively, down the phone to my ex-husband and, as a bonus, get a long letter from Caitlin and Richard saying that they are moving out.

I'll have to sell the house now, no choice. My mind is in chaos, which makes it hard to learn my lines for Montréal. There is no space or peace in my brain for them to lodge in. The night before I leave for Montréal Lise, who has worked for me for fourteen years, faxes me her notice to quit. This bad luck is inexorable. I feel bludgeoned by events. I am now

165

convinced that there is more afoot than I can see. I take my sleeping pills but sleep evades me all night long. There is not one second of respite from the churning thoughts. In desperation I get up and begin to make lists of what I'll need in the new flat, what I'll have to sell or dump. It just makes bad worse.

I leave St Louis in a sad state. I dread the flight as we leave in a thunderstorm and there is no alcohol aboard an internal American flight. I change planes in Chicago, but I am so exhausted I sleep. Unbelievable. I sleep on a plane. When I wake I have lines to learn. I have lines to learn. I am so ecstatic at being back in professional harness that the next two days pass in a euphoria of work.

The 'talk', illustrated with bits of acted Shakespeare, goes very well indeed, especially after I have explained the reason for my shortness of temper to the stage manager from the production company who is staging this conference. Even in my strung-out state, I realise they know a lot about conferences and nothing about theatre. Of course, the wide, carpeted ballroom of the Hilton Hotel in Montréal in no way resembles a theatre, and it's a blessing to be miked against its engulfing wall and floor padding that sucks in most sound and muffles what's left. It's normally considered an insult to mike classical actors. Afterwards, Professor Andy Gurr from the Globe, who preceded me with a brilliant

166

illustrated lecture of the history of the Globe theatres, and I retreat, to congratulate ourselves and each other, to a little French restaurant I ate in by chance some—it takes me a while and many fingers to work it out—some thirty-two years ago when I was last in Canada, with Sir Laurence Olivier's National Theatre company. It is bizarre, this synchronicity and bending of time. More so when the owner insists he remembers the previous visit.

The following morning, having rerun the show most of the night in my aching, disoriented head, I decide to sightsee Montréal before a good long afternoon rest. My flight leaves early in the evening. No having to check out here on the morning of departure, as we do in the penny-pinching theatre: this is the world of corporate business and first-class air travel. I walk the streets of the city in as alert a manner as my physical frailty and zombied brain will allow. The warmth of the sun spreads into my grateful back. I do manage to recall certain buildings in Old Montréal. So it *is* my brain that's inside my skull. I ask directions for *la rivière*, which elicits odd looks from an elegant lady with sculpted black hair and dark red lips who reminds me eerily of my mother. 'La fleuve?' she corrects me, then asks, because my accent is devoid of the Canadian nasal twang, 'Vous êtes de Paris?' as they did last time I was here, which is a comfort, and, like last time, I reply, 'Non, Madame, de Londres.' I stand facing the wind where the fast flowing St Lawrence joins the Ottawa river, feeling the breeze blowing through my very bones, clearing out the two days of stuffy air from planes and hotel rooms. Having stopped, I realise how far I've walked, how much I ache, how tired I am, find it hard to get started again, but decide that on my return walk I will go and sit in the cathedral for a rest. I could do with enlisting some help for what I have to face in England. Oh, and a quick thank-you to my much overworked guardian angels for allowing me to scrape through the texts without, as far as I can recall, a mistake wouldn't go amiss either. As I approach the imposing centre doors of the cathedral, slowly, by an unseen hand, they open, and there in front of me, barring my way, complete with ornamental brass fittings, is a large white coffin.

CHAPTER NINE

Up but Not Away

I am so excited by flying first class, for only the second time in my life, and not wanting to waste this experience of luxury—the seat extends into a full-length bed—and as there are only two or three businessmen in the whole of the cabin, all asleep—the air hostesses, when they're not fussing over me, and I spend most of the journey chatting.

When I land at Heathrow I feel as if I am not part of the world at all. My friend Patricia has driven from Warwickshire to meet me. She scoops me up in a huge hug and takes me back to the cottage. It's our first real chance to be together, and we talk all the way. She had badly wanted to come to Paris to see me too. I am elated by her kindness and overjoyed by the welcome and the lunch next door. Disconcertingly the ground keeps swaying up to meet me. It's hard to know what is jet-lag and what is brain-fag. When I finally admit to being beaten by the time, the wine and the fatigue, reluctantly I retreat to the cottage. The phone rings. It's Ann. She tells me succinctly, not a syllable to spare, that much-loved Joe W died this morning. The timing is deplorable. Joe W (Audrey's husband) was a childhood icon of my son's. He wore yellow sweaters and brown cord trousers. He was a big gentle bear of a man. My son called him Winnie the Pooh.

I wander aimlessly through the rooms. My mind is adrift. I feel bludgeoned and beaten by loss. I am afloat, unanchored, wrong. In bed I hear cries. There is little release. Days pass. Nights stick. I am astray. I think, Hold on to the sides. I am capsized.

I must get out. I must Get On. I must. I tout around for a bike to borrow. Patricia has one. Ironically it has a curved cross-bar, just like the one I used to ride as a teenager. Some cheap, embarrassing old bone-shaker of a bike that someone threw out, or didn't want, which ended up with us. My foster-mother and I were often the recipients of people's pity and slightly scuffed shoes. How I hated that bike's curved cross-bar. How it shamed me. The sit-up-and-beg handlebars. This one, in one of Patricia's outhouses, is identical. I feel nothing but love for it. I borrow it, christen it Miss Plum—it is maroon—buy a basket for its front and buy a helmet for my head. Wearing it feels a bit pathetic. Shutting the stable door after the brain has bolted. At least I can get out and about on my own. Do my own shopping. I remember how riding a bike to grammar school felt. How the wind sang in my ears. How free and jubilant I felt. Now I teeter down the country lanes, feeling as if the wheels are caught in resistant chewing-gum.

At least, I placate myself, as I struggle to complete each circuit of the pedals, I can do my own shopping. That's what this acute expenditure of energy is about. Revelling in my freedom, I binge with choice and come back with a bicycle laden like a tinker's moll. I have to get off and push it up even the slightest incline. Inclines that aren't there in a car. Even on the flat bits, when I've managed to get up a little steam, there is a risk that the unbalanced loads will suddenly make the bike veer off sharply in any direction. I am frightened of falling, as never before. There is a humming in my ears from exertion, and the pounding of my heart thuds alarmingly in my chest, but in spite of exhaustion, I am a shred resembling jubilant.

That night I find it hard to focus on the red knitting. The stitches blur and double in front of my tired eyes. The scarf has grown like a long red gash. I measure it against myself. It is almost as tall as I am.

I have to get some money. The little pension isn't enough. I'll have to sell the house. I have to go to London to sell the house. I have to face the demons. I have to visit the neuro-surgeon. I have to have an EEG test. (I have no idea at the time that all these haves are to stop me feeling have-nots.)

I have to go to London on my own. Who else is there? The idea terrifies me. The notion of being in London is full of terrors. As it turns out, there are demons in store for me long before I get there.

It is a sweltering day. Usually I rejoice in the sun. Today the light settles in a tight band across my eyes and I resent it. The train is late. The train is full. I cannot stand all the way to London, I am simply not able to. I hurry, as much as I can, towards the last empty seat in a carriage. I manage to get there just before a young woman. She is being shielded solicitously by a young man, who states, 'Let my wife sit down, she's pregnant.'

I scan her. There is no visible bump on the young woman's stomach. Precipitous proud father-to-be. I hear a querulous, irascible voice say, in a one-upmanship sort of way, 'I've had brain surgery.' I feel all the eyes in the carriage scan my scarless red face.

I spend a hot, uncomfortable journey, holding my head as the train careers from side to side. This is not solely for the benefit of my brain, which is sloshing about inside my skull. I want anyone who still happens to be looking at me to know how very bad I feel. I feel red and raw, inside and out. Every bump in the track, every bend of the way exerts a different sense of tightness in my brain. I take exception to the set of that woman's mouth. I loathe the busy pattern on that man's pullover. That couple look dumb enough to be ideally suited. That child across the gangway is ugly and looks stupid. It gazes at me quizzically. I want to scream and make it jump. It offends me. I glance away, deciding it is too despicable for my regard. To take my mind off inside, I look outside.

I am stopped in trying to demonstrate how bad I feel by how bad I feel. I try to concentrate on the book I have brought with

172

me, but I can't get comfortable, neither inside nor out. I've never liked Trollope and *The Warden* hangs heavy on my fragile interest. It is my twenty-seventh book this year. Well, twenty-six and a half. I know I won't finish it. I look around the carriage again. I used to like people in a sort of vague, ineffectual way. I always felt the human race was basically sort of all right. Now I hate everyone I see. I actively loathe them. Everyone, without exception, looks gross, grotesque: eyes too close together, a huge jaw, a twisted stoop, a lazy slouch. I am appalled at the utter ugliness of the human race. Who am I?

When we arrive at Paddington I have trouble standing up. I lose my balance when I do manage it. Or, rather, I can't find my balance in the first place. My brain is still moving in motion with the train, but my body is stationary. And somewhere I—whoever that is—am trying to make sense of these two disparate bits. I am hot and sticky and bad-tempered. I want to push everyone out of the way. I feel so cramped, so robbed of air. The closeness of the other bodies in the queue for the door feels like an invasion of the worst kind. I must have space. I want to push an old lady out of the way, she's taking too long. I can't stand not moving. I can't stand standing. A young girl's rucksack catches my shoulder as she turns round to pick her things off the table. I exert pressure against it. Quite consciously and deliberately I push back against it. She turns and stares at me. I glare back at her. Don't they know I've been ill? They must let me off first. I have been very ill. The queue straggles along slowly, my frustration and impatience growing. Assessing the gap between the step and the platform is hard. I wave my right foot tentatively in the direction of what I perceive as the space, which is unaccountably and intriguingly far away, when it comes smack up against something hard. The platform. How odd, but I have no time to muse about the discrepancy between my eyes and my foot as the surge of people rushing along the platform from further up the train threatens to topple me. As I whip my head round to monitor them, my brain actually makes a zapping noise. A small angry wasp is caught in my neck. I look behind at the queue of people in my wake. Did they hear it? I am met by sullen stares. Their irritation with my slowness is tangible. I can feel it in the noisome, torrid air. Again the wasp makes a short sharp snarl. I force myself into the abyss and, although I end up jarring my spine and jolting my head, I have managed to get two feet on the platform. I moan out loud at the sight of the swarms of people coming from the opposite direction towards me. I will have to walk through them to get to the tube. As each person passes me, I flinch mentally. I moan out loud again. Neat. Several people hear and give me a wide berth.

No *need* to act mad.

The tube is the worst nightmare I have ever had. The worst kind of hell. I am as unstable as a cork tossed this way and that. Up stairs full of people, down corridors full of people. I am jostled and pushed by unseen currents and cross-currents. At last on a platform, I force myself to walk the length of it to find a vacant seat and sit, with my head in my hands, till the train roars into the station. It's a fight to get on. I have to keep my eyes closed so I can't see how near people are. Spitefully, I push against the briefcase that's edging into the back of my knees. 'Can you get your bag out of my legs?' I create a pool of discomfort around me by asking the unaskable. I don't care. I elbow the umbrella handle that's threatening to lodge itself in my shoulder. As the tube lurches from side to side I can't seem to manage to stand on two feet at the same time. It never crosses my dazed mind to ask if I can sit down.

I am glad to be home. I am surprised I am glad to be home. It feels strangely luxurious with its fitted carpets, after the rather Spartan nature and the flagstone floor of the cottage. It seems so new and fresh, although I have lived here for twenty years. It is, after all, a home, not rented accommodation. It's full of memories from little things garnered over the years. I've never been an acquisitive person, and these

175

little objects—a small flower vase with end-of-the-week multi-coloured glaze splashes all over it, a little pottery milk jug covered in flowers from Capri, a mosaic photo frame from Venice, a round pebble of bright Bristol blue glass from my theatre club in Bristol, a small starfish from among the shingle at Aldeburgh, a framed Victorian map of Suffolk—are all valueless except for the significance they hold for me, the memory of the day and the way they came into my life. That significance seems inexplicably deeper now. The memories are proof, I realise slowly, that that bit of my brain is working. That, too, is a comfort.

'We are our memories,' says my son, when the subject crops up later in conversation on the telephone.

'I think we are our choices,' I argue. I argue easily these days. 'And if we are the choices we make, then who are we when we have no choice?' I'm full of smart-alec thoughts like this too. I'm thinking of the humiliating, humbling lack of choice in Intensive Care.

'No, I think it's memories,' he insists. I want to shake him till his teeth rattle.

I wish I didn't feel so glad to be home. It makes it harder to say goodbye and trudge the streets looking for somewhere else. But I have to. I need the money. How long will it be before I can work again full-time? is the unasked question. The question I don't have the guts to ask myself. So I have to sell. In

176

spite of the kindness of the RSC and the Royal Theatrical Fund, whose unsolicited generosity made me cry when I saw the cheques, I have to move. It wasn't just the money and the relief from worry they brought, it was the acknowledgement of my work that came with it. Work. My spirits start on a downward spiral. As if on cue with the dawnings of regret, a sledgehammer starts banging the wall next door, making the ornaments and pictures on my mantelpiece tremble and jump.

I gasp at the noise, grab the front-door keys and charge out. Risking losing my balance on the muddy planks that are bridging the front doorstep I burst into what used to be Glad's neatly polished living room, with its patterned rugs and floral cushions, and scream at the two young men who are sledgehammering the plaster off the walls. 'Stop it! Stop it! I'm recovering from brain surgery! The noise hurts! Stop it!'

They stare at me as if I am mad. They attempt to burble explanations, but I will have none of it. I am past flashpoint and shaking with the exertions of shouting. I am also overcome to see dear old Glad's house in this totally wrecked state, although she, with Alzheimer's in a geriatric ward, is thankfully out of it in every sense. I stumble back next door, trying to hide the cascading snot and tears. Well, I think, trying to master the situation, there's another reason to move now.

177

CHAPTER TEN

Down and Out of It

But mastery won't come. Nothing comes. I don't know what I'm feeling, what to feel. I don't know whether to feel glad or sad but, then, that's nothing unusual, these days. The thumping and hammering punctuate the rest of my time in the house. How could I have forgotten they are refurbishing next door? It had started BC, before I went to Paris. Extraordinary that they are still not finished. Such a great gap of time seems to have gone by.

The builders and their accompaniment of blaring pop music arrive with reliable regularity every morning, dead on the dot of half past seven, and at eight o'clock exactly the hammering begins. There is no comfort, but an odd kind of symmetry in the thumps that are happening both inside and outside my head. I snarl and occasionally shout back at the noise. I feel like the porter in *Macbeth*.

The bedroom smells strange. I open all the windows and light candles in several rooms, which makes me feel better. But the smell persists. What can it be?

I check my shoes for dog shit.

No.

It must be the shit in my mind.

I double up on the sleeping pills, not out of fear. Yes, out of fear. Fear of a bad smell? Get a grip. But no grip is to be got. I rationalise the dawning awareness that the more overtired I become the more sleep evades me. I hit it with the chemical hammer. Then, eventually, sleep comes. I wake in my own bed without the vaguest notion of where I am. The distant rattle of the District Line starting up reminds me. It must be about half past four.

Light is leaking under the curtains. I don't like being here alone any more. I finger the scar. That has become the touchstone of why I am where I am. Oh, yes. Scar. Ill. Need money. Sell house.

Darleney and I meet. We walk. Well, she walks, I go like a crab. We see the dream flat. It's exactly what I want and where I want it. She encourages me to sit down on the sofa and just 'get the feel of the room', but I know she has seen me shaking. It's only on the first floor, but I could barely manage the stairs. She offered a discreet hand under my elbow at one point. I am shocked that she can see how frail I am. I stare about me, vague and pleased to be wherever it is we are. It is a pleasant large room. The place has a good feel to it. Not that I can trust what I feel, these days, I remind whichever of the selves is listening.

She suggests I put in an offer for it. I have no idea what she is talking about. 'The flat, you like it, don't you?'

'Oh, yes, it's lovely.'

'You would like it, wouldn't you?'

Again this feeling of being a child. I want to nod and say, 'Yes, please.' Yes, please. Buy me this lollipop, and it will all be done. I look around again. The big bay windows let in a lot of light. I'll need a large oblong table right across that width to work on and to sit friends round to eat. I don't have a large oblong table. The curtains are too dark: I would change them to light-coloured ones. I would have to make them because of the expense of made-to-measure. Where is my sewing-machine? I can't remember where it is. It seems very important that I locate it. I feel my lower lip tremble and the back of my throat start to sting. This is ridiculous. I am ridiculous. The sewing-machine is at Ann's. I never got round to using it. All the sewing I did for her there was by hand. I must get it back. I stifle an overpowering desire to ring her there and then and demand the return of the sewing-machine. I am suddenly boiling. I can feel the sweat running down the sides of my grimy face into my grimy neck. I pat at it ineffectually. I feel very dirty. Like the London-stained windows. Beyond the dirt, the windows are full of the leaves of the trees in the park across the road.

In the winter when I'm here, if I'm here—if I'm alive, of course—when I'm alive, if I'm here, those trees will be bare, of course. Bare. Empty. For a few blissful seconds, the twister that is my mind is empty too.

'What does the traffic sound like?' I ask. The estate agent looks at us in a curious way. Or is it me? Is he looking at me? What did I say?

'I can't hear it,' Darleney answers.

'Well, that's all right, then, isn't it?' But it isn't. The estate agent casts me another glance. I want to say, 'You think I'm weird? *I* think I'm weird. You should be in my shoes.'

I want to take my shoes off my hot, aching, swollen feet and burrow into the sofa and never move, ever. I want Darleney to tuck me up and bring me glasses with ice in to drink and put her cool hands on my forehead and stay by me.

We have coffee in a nearby square, to which I walk with great difficulty in spite of hanging on to her arm. 'Oh, I can see you living there, Janie,' she says, in her gentle, encouraging way, patting my hand as we move apart to our separate chairs. I lean my arms heavily on the table, grateful to be sitting down at last. I don't want to do anything except place my head on its cool metal surface. Every car whizzing by is like a lash across my face. I look around, astonished that no one at the other tables is remarking on the noise of the constant traffic.

181

I can't see myself living anywhere. I'm not even glad to be alive. I want the noise to stop and the dull ache in my head to go away. I want to crawl home to bed. Home. I want to go home. And Darleney must come with me, of course. She just must.

When we get home Darleney suggests I ring my solicitor. I cannot believe that she has suggested this. Doesn't she know how I feel? I ring my solicitor, garble the details, get them wrong, have to ask Darleney, have to write them down in the notebook I carry with me all the time now, and try again. The numbers make no sense. Perhaps they do, but what's left of my mind can't accept it. It is an outlandish sum of money. It is an overwhelming amount. What I mean is, just thinking about the amount of money overwhelms me. Then I realise that every object I can see just in this room, the sitting room, will have to have three decisions made about it. Chuck it? Keep it? Give it away? The enormity makes me cry. Then I feel ridiculous that I am crying over such a thing because the old me would have had no trouble in dealing with this by making several lists. Then lists of lists. Then I realise I don't know who this person is who can't cope. I always cope. I have coped since my foster-mother sent me into the town on a trolley-bus of a Saturday morning aged twelve to pay the rates.

That felt so wrong. So does this. Coping is my thing. I can't cope with not coping. I feel as if I am going mad. I hear a Grace Poole cackle in the east wing.

The next day the phone rings with the offer of the summer teaching job I usually do in Oxford. It means four half-days of work with a one-day break in the middle. That seems reasonable enough. As I am accepting it, I promise myself I will go to bed early in college each night, having bought my regular supply of food, to save me the shattering noise of a hundred and fifty students in the vast refectory. They are pleased that I will work for them again, finding actors to teach is always a precarious and last-minute business, but they voice anxiety about whether I will be able to manage it. I pooh-pooh their concern. I explain I've already done a masterclass and two charity shows in St Louis, a Shakespeare demonstration for the Globe in Montréal, and I'm going to do a recital of Victorian poetry with two good friends in Stratford in the summer. I feel slightly guilty about this recital as apart from the initial reading, during which I realised I didn't like any of the poems, I haven't given the script a further thought. So I *have* to do this teaching job. If I don't, they might not offer it to me again. And teaching work is the one oasis of surety in what might be a desert of a year in acting jobs, especially if the news gets round that I am—was—ill. I must work this year to prepare for and confirm the next. That seems perfectly logical and reasonable to me. A perfectly logical and reasonable little voice says, 'But you might not be here next year.' I choose to ignore it. Weighing heavy in my bag, and adding to the irony, Darleney has given me a hardback copy of Will Self's *How the Dead Live.* I say, 'I should know.'

A woman bumps into me in the newsagent's on Paddington station and says, 'I'm sorry.'

'No, you're not,' I say.

'What?' she says.

'You're not sorry. You're not sorry at all,' I say. 'I don't know why people utter such meaningless nonsense.'

She gives me a peculiar look and hurries off.

I decide to buy some soup from the stall on the station, I often do. Did. Used to. It helps fill the time till the train comes. I also realise that I can't remember where or when I had my last meal. Or what it was. Two young American students are serving. The girl says, 'Yes?'

'Tomato and basil.'

'Tomayto and bay-zil,' she says to the boy, who must have heard what I said perfectly well. It's a status thing. 'Bread?'

'No, thank you. I can't eat bread. I have a wheat allergy. Wheat makes me ill.'

The boy says, 'Small, regular or large?'

'Large, please. I don't think I've eaten all day. It's interesting how the use of the word "regular" has crept into the English language. I mean over here, in England. From America. I teach in America. In fact, I've not long been back from Wash U.' I use the shorthand version so they will know I know America. 'You guys are very quiet,' I continue, 'you must have been over here too long. You're getting Anglicised—you're becoming English.' I laugh. I think of how outspoken the Americans are in comparison to the English. There is the faintest smile playing around the boy's mouth. I smile back.

The girl hands me the soup in a little brown carrier-bag and says, 'Don't you *ever* stop talking?'

I am stung. I don't know what to say.

'I've been ill. Very ill,' I mumble, abashed. When I pick up the bag and turn to walk away, the woman waiting in the queue behind me, whom I didn't know was there, won't meet my eye.

On the train I find a seat. I take the soup out of the bag, put it on the little ledge beside me, and settle down to the idea of enjoying it and it doing me good. A much-needed gesture of self-care. A young man comes and sits opposite. As he settles himself down he catches the carton and boiling hot soup goes all over the floor and me. My feet are scalded. I take the newspaper that is lying on the seat

185

and make an attempt to soak up the excess. The floor is awash with orange liquid. My black sandals are streaked with fibres of tomato but I can't ignore that my red varnished toes look quite at home in their colourful surroundings. 'Go and ask one of the train staff to bring a cloth to wipe it up,' I say. I see from his blank look that he doesn't speak much English. 'Ask—help—train,' I say louder, in the best English-tourist-abroad manner. He gets up to go, taking his bags with him.

'You won't see him again,' says the woman sitting opposite me on the other side of the gangway.

'That's a very cynical view of human nature,' I say, surprised at her interjection and even more surprised by the speed of my own optimistic response. (Snake that I was on my way down to town.)

'I'd put money on it,' she continues.

The young man doesn't come back.

On days when the sun is out I sit in the garden at the cottage drinking far too much wine, hoping it will blank out the endless chatter in my head. I look through the poems for the recital in a desultory manner. The pages reflect the sun: they are almost unbearably white. I look away. There are so many greens in the leaves of the plants. The blue-tinged nettles with a fine coating of dust on their saw-toothed edges, the yellow and light green mottled leaves of the privet shoots, the dark, shiny smoothness of those on the periwinkle. It's almost impossible to keep my attention on Tennyson or Swinburne when so many colours are jumping out at me and demanding to be seen. Then a brainwave hits me. I will learn a poem a day. That will damn well stop the chatter in my head or, at least, give me a better class of burble. How much memory have I lost exactly? Recalling the Shakespeare in St Louis and Montréal was relatively easy. That's comforting. Let's see how my new brain copes with new stuff. What's more, I think, warming to my theme, I won't allow myself to look at the shopping list when I go to the village shop either. I'll learn the damn list too.

I start for good measure with Gerard Manley Hopkins. If my new brain can retain *that* then I'm—what?

Ready for work? I'm—what? I'm all right? I'm—

The world is charged with the grandeur of
    God.
It will flame out like shining from shook
    foil . . .
It gathers to a greatness, like the ooze of oil
Crushed. Why do men then now not reck
    his rod?

187

Generations have trod, have trod, have
  trod;
And all is seared with trade; bleared,
  smeared with toil;
And wears man's smudge and shares man's
  smell—

That takes me all day. Eight lines takes me all
day. My mind keeps wandering off. Not so
much a bucking bronco, more like an elusive
strip of mist. Each time I think I've caught it—
that I'm concentrating—I open my hand to
find it's empty, that my attention has drifted
into something quite other. I can recall most of
the first verse the next morning, though. I walk
to the village shop saying it. I skip down the
road in the sunshine like a schoolgirl. Once
there, I count off the five items from the
learned list on my fingers. 'Three began with
C,' I say. Cake, (wheat-free), Cleaner (for loo)
and Cards (for friends), something with B and
some stamps. What was the B? What *was* it?

'Oh, you should write a list,' says a helpful
shop assistant, from behind the counter.

'I've got one in my bag,' I reply defensively.
'What *was* the B?' I ask the world at large,
refusing to consult my list. I smile at the two
people in the queue. The blowsy, untidy
woman, with stains on her T-shirt and hair
awry, stares directly at me, and a man in a
trilby, green waistcoat and tie pretends he
hasn't been watching me and looks intently at

the chocolate bars on the counter as I catch his eye. The village shop caters for both ends of the social scale. I know which response I prefer. I favour the brazen stare. It's more honest.

'B . . .? B . . .? Oh, bugger it,' I say, to no one in particular. The atmosphere in the shop is frostier than the fridge.

When the sun moves from the cottage back garden over the neighbour's roof, I take all my papers and books and sit in the garden at the front. The sun beats down. It is very hot. Underneath my hat, my scalp itches and itches. I scratch it until the skin breaks. There are slight smears of blood on my fingers, but there is no relief. A friend passes. 'Don't go overdoing it in the sun,' she says kindly.

'If we only did what was allowed, we'd all be sitting in cardboard boxes,' I snap back. She goes on walking up the hill. What is wrong with me?

Nights pass when the chatter in my head doesn't let up for a second. One sleeping tablet. I read till three in the morning, till my eyes smart and won't focus any more. Easy to be absorbed. I'm reading Coetzee's brilliant *Disgrace*. Book number twenty-seven. Another sleeping tablet. Still the endless replay of scenes from hospital life goes on behind my eyes, even when they're closed. At night I have nothing to think about except all the things that have gone wrong and how awful my body feels. Another sleeping tablet. I want to bang my head against the wall. I seriously consider doing it and, wondering whether the titanium clip would fall off if I did, I fall asleep.

I so long for silence in my head that a grudge begins to grow when I'm in the one place where I feel silence ought to be provided and isn't—church. The number of words that I can't and won't say has grown in proportion to the resentment. Patricia calls in on her way up the hill one afternoon, waking me up in the garden from a rare *al fresco* snooze, and I strike out at everyone and everything that makes me angry—the list is long and church is included. It comes in for more than the lion's share of derision. She's often thought of going to Quakers, she tells me, her family in Northumberland were Quaker. I recall how I enjoyed my times at Quaker meetings in St Louis. I jump at the suggestion and pin her down to a time to meet and go. The speed and urgency of my decision surprises both of us.

The silence of the meeting house is balm to my soul. Centuries of peace unfurl from the walls and engulf me. It is easier to discard thought in the healing comfort of other people's quiet. I am filled with gratitude for the peaceful figures around me.

It's been such a long time since I've felt anything resembling affection for the human race that in turn I feel the dawning of a rare small shred of self-liking too. I am just sinking down into the space, leaving the chattering nonsense behind, when Patricia squeezes my hand. It is a loving, kindly gesture, it makes me open my eyes. I want to kill her. Nice notion in a Friends' meeting house.

Later, in the car going home, she tells me that I spoke out during the coffee break after the meeting in a way that I wouldn't have before I was ill. I am shocked. She knows something about me that I don't—a childhood bomb button. As a child I was often conscious that the world knew the secret of why my mother didn't want me, why she walked away from me when I was two months old, but that I never would know. My fury at Patricia grows. But I am brought up sharp by realising that as I am living alone there is no one to monitor my behaviour in this way or compare it with what went before. A flash of realisation. But the old fury wins out against any burgeoning gratitude. 'You're much harder on other people since you've been ill,' she says. I battle with myself to swallow back the justification for my dislike. 'And you're much harder on yourself too.' Then I know I'm lucky to have her as a friend. I must remember to be grateful for her care. How long will she stay the course, I wonder, whatever the course now is?

191

CHAPTER ELEVEN

Help!

One morning the cottage phone rings just as I'm about to settle myself to some more poem learning, indoors as it's so grey outside. The dream flat's gone: it's been snapped up by someone who has nothing to sell. I am crestfallen. It was mine. It was. It was perfect. Darleney and I are back to square one in the flat-hunting scene. I must find a new home. I must have a new home because I have a new life. I must.

Several demanding calls later, especially when put on hold and my head's blasted by deafeningly loud, insulting music, I end by shouting down the phone to the non-listening air. I have managed to fit in three appointments in London in two days. I also have a dull throb in my head, and have tangled badly with the neuro-surgeon's receptionist. I get times and dates muddled: 'I would have thought you, of all people, would have made allowances for brain patients,' I say, still astride my high horse. If people whose job is dealing with the brain-damaged don't make allowances . . . I can't quite put my finger on how the tangle occurred. When tired (and the phone tires me almost more quickly than anything else), my brain alights on the first fact going and runs with it. Anyhow, I have now run out of preposterousness . . . Nevertheless I've wangled an appointment with the neuro-surgeon of my choice, who dealt with my driving licence.

More flats are lined up for me and Darleney to view—or, rather, for her to assess and tell me what to think. Lastly I've arranged a visit to my gynaecologist to address yet another physical problem I've had for some time. I have started bleeding intermittently because the hospital didn't know I was on HRT when I was in Intensive Care, so my whole cycle, or what's left of it at fifty-five, is shot to pieces— or at least has decided to have its two penn'orth of medical attention too. Peter, a kindly neighbour, drives me to the station on another blazing hot day. 'You'll cook in London,' he says ruefully. I do. I fry and bake, and let off a lot of steam.

Home. I try to block out the sense of other people having walked through my home. It feels different, though the pile of junk mail is, almost comfortingly, the same in both garishness and amount. I have trouble getting the front door open through it. The garden is mightily overgrown. The Virginia creeper at the back has slithered all over the walls and the roof of the bathroom, and long fingers of it hang down past the sitting-room window. It is like a house that has slept for a hundred years. The time warp feels apt. At the front the curly fronds of wisteria wave in the breeze, like tentacles that are curious to test the space. The jasmine has shot out gawky long stalks above the hedge line, and the ancient white rose that creeps through it is covered with greenfly.

I do what I always do when I get back to London after being away: get the step-ladder and the electric hedge-trimmer and perch precariously on the uneven ground at the front, wielding the saw at the offending greenery. When I switch it on, the sound it makes is terrifying. I jump and nearly unbalance myself. It must be done. The house must look tidy or it'll never sell. By the time it looks even vaguely neat, I've two black bags full of trimmings, old leaves and sweet wrappers, which get tossed by the wind under the fence, and the odd cola can that gets thrown over it. Sweat is trickling down my neck and face, my hair is stuck to my head under my hat and my T-shirt has wet stains front and back. I tidy things away and catch a glimpse of the clock: I have half an hour to wash and get to the neuro-surgeon. I can't rush. To rush is to feel ill. As it is, I am shaking with exhaustion. Where has the afternoon gone? What is the matter with me? All I've done is catch a damn train, get to London and

194

trim the garden.

The neuro-surgeon, let's call him Mr Y, has all the Rolls-Royce attributes of the brain surgeon. Softly spoken, luxurious office, Mont Blanc pen. He is not the man I remember seeing two, three years ago. Why should that surprise me? Nothing is the same. It is all new. I am here at Parkside Hospital to find out what to do.

'Neurontin? You don't need to be on that if you haven't had a fit.'

'Well . . . I had one when I collapsed.'

'Yes, but that's just part of the haemorrhage. We'll get you off that slowly.'

'What if I have a fit?'

Then we'll put you back on it. Or something like it.'

'And an EEG?'

'Well, that won't tell us much.'

'They said in France—'

'They would, they're very fond of EEG.'

'They said I should have another MRI scan too.' *Did* they? I think. Or was it the *American* brain surgeon who said that?

'When did you have your last one?'

'Er . . . My last what?' I have no idea what he's just said. All I can think of is the dull ache in my lower back. Damn electric hedge-trimmer. I want to scratch and scratch my head. Actually, to be more precise, I want to bang it against the wall.

'Do you have trouble with your memory?'

'Will I? I mean, if I have no memory I have no job.'

'You'll probably be able to recall stuff you'd learned before the aneurysm burst, but new stuff . . .'

Gerard Manley Hopkins, I think, Ha, ha. I find enough strength in that to ask, 'What did you just ask me?'

'MRI scan. They put you in a tunnel—'

'Oh, I remember *that.* The terrible noise.' I don't mean it to come out as a criticism but it does. I think that because I see him stiffen slightly. I add lamely, 'Marvellous machines—I don't mind the noise at all.' Obsequious snake. Me. Not him.

'So, when?'

'Wh-wh-when . . .?' I notice that I have begun to slur my words.

'MRI scan?'

'Er, March. March the seventeenth.' Triumph. I wait for him to be impressed.

'Well, you don't need another so soon.'

'But I—'

'My dear girl.' I have never been able to tolerate men who my-dear-girl me. 'Do you know my brother-in-law? He's in the business.'

'What name of?' Why am I not making sense?

He says something along the lines of 'John Brown.'

'What?' I am lost.

'He was in that play with—oh, you know, what's her name? She always does those West End kind of comedies.'

'Zena Dare? Faith Brown? Nyree Dawn Porter? Dinah Sheridan?'

He shakes his head after each name. Aren't I supposed to be thinking of men? I think.

'Anyway, I think Dinah Sheridan's dead.'

'I . . . I have a second aneurysm.'

'Statistically, the chances of you having a second—'

I feel my throat begin to sting and constrict. 'But I do . . . They told me at the hospital—'

'Which hospital?'

'Um . . . er. The hospital in Paris—where they saved my life.' I feel such a loyalty I have to say this. Though I think it probably unwise to remind him of someone else's skill. Why? It feels like he could do without it. I don't see him stiffen now. I *feel* it. I'm keen to changes in atmosphere. Like when I was a child and I could always sense the unspoken war between my foster-mother and my real mother on the few occasions my real mother turned up and tried to get me back. But I still can't recall the name. There's a blank where the hospital's name ought to be. I was there for a month, for goodness' sake. This is bad. I can learn poems, though, I remonstrate with myself defensively. Gerard Manley Hopkins, what's more. I suspect this would be lost on *him*, though.

Him? Mr Neuro-surgeon. Who? Him. Here. What? Hospital. Yes. Where? Paris. I want to say, 'It's near the Gare du Nord. My son used to get off the train and walk through to the hospital.' My eyes fill with tears. Why? I don't know why. What were we talking about? I don't know what to think. Then I think, It's in the papers. He's got the papers. He's had the papers for three months.

'It must be in there.' There is a tinge of desperation. I can hear it in my voice. I point to the file with my name on it on his desk. My hand is shaking.

'My goodness, you do get worked up easily!'

Something snaps inside me. I hear it. 'Yes, well, I've had brain surgery.'

My tone surprises even him. 'You're very emotional, aren't you?'

'Yes, that's why I'm an actor and not an accountant.' I have no idea who this person is who's answering in my place. I need help. Help. Yes. 'Is there a support group?' I try to temper what's been said by asking this mildly and pseudo-sweetly. I despise myself for it.

'What?'

'A support group.' I think of the American brain surgeon and the papers his office sent me to read. The information about the support group was on top of the pile. For some ridiculous reason the word 'support' echoes round my brain and tears splash down from somewhere.

'I have no idea.' The implication is that my question is absurd and directed at the wrong person. 'Now, we all have to face death—'

A dull ache is beginning to make itself felt at the base of my skull. 'I've faced it, Mr Y, have you?' I can't believe I said that. I point again, irritated, at the file. 'It's hot. I'm tired.'

'I'm hot and I'm tired too.'

He answers, I think, childishly. You have no bloody right to be tired, you're a doctor, for Christ's sake, you're *in charge*, I want to scream.

He riffles through the papers. 'Statistically—'

'I'm not a statistic, I'm a person.' I say it like I know who I'm talking about. At least the anger is out in the open. Whoever it comes from.

'Oh, ye-es,' he says slowly, deflecting my anger, as he finds the relevant image and holds it up to the light before putting it on the white screen behind him. I don't want to see it. I turn away, like a child refusing to eat. What *do* I want? Why am I here? Well, somebody's got to look after me in England.

'Can you see the second aneurysm?' I ask petulantly, wanting to rub his nose in it.

He brushes aside what I've said, by saying smoothly, 'You'll probably die of breast cancer before the second aneurysm gets you.'

I sit outside in the reception area waiting for a

199

minicab, heaving. The world is a terrible place.

He walks past to get into his expensive car. 'Has somebody rung for a cab for you?' he asks, almost concerned. I barely nod, thinking, Your concern is too little and too late. Somebody has to look after me, yes, and it's not you.

My son arrives late in a black cab and I do the one thing I know I mustn't. I dissolve.

CHAPTER TWELVE

Round and Round I Go

The London night is oppressive and very noisy. It stretches like elastic. I sleep in fits and starts. I have a dream that stays with me for several days. Two lions are side by side. One is old and mangy, careworn and moth-eaten, though there is still pride in his bearing. The other is a young cub who sits dutifully and calmly by him. I don't know why the dream feels so significant and resonant, but it does. I can recall it at will. It also catches me by surprise by turning up spontaneously at odd times.

I call the estate agent the next morning and ask him not to bring anyone round as I'm at home. He asks if he can pop in for the briefest moment as he has some papers he wants me to sign. When the doorbell goes I am, thankfully, near enough to hear it, but when I open the door, although I've met him several times before, I have no idea who he is. I am unnerved when he says his name.

The District Line in a heatwave is a terrible place, especially when it decides to go no further than Earl's Court. I will be late for the gynaecologist. Late. Panic. No actor is ever late. That's drummed into you from day one at drama school. I run to get on the first bus I see. It goes to the Marylebone Road. I settle in, pleased and proud. It's not the tube. I have a view. I begin to look out of the window with real interest. I should use buses more. This is a great way of travelling, although it does bump my head a bit. I try to rest it on the coolness of the window, but that bumps it even more. A woman gets on at the next stop and sits next to me. I resent everything about her: the way she looks, her arm, which rests near mine, her dyed hair (I have dyed hair) and, to top it all, she smiles at me in a placatory way as she senses, rightly, that I am trying to edge as far away from her as I can. To make matters worse I see now she is Indian. Well, I can't stop now. She's in my space. I manage, by leaning into the window and turning away from her, to remove almost all of my body from any contact with her whatsoever. This is

201

my space, damn it. At her every involuntary touch, my body flares with exasperation and my brain with ill-will.

The bus corners badly and she drops some of the parcels she is carrying into the aisle. I daren't help her. There's a step between her bags and the front seat that we're perched on and when I look down, my sense of balance goes and I risk hitting my head against the panelling that separates us from the steeply curving stairs. As she retrieves her packages and straightens up in her seat, she is no longer smiling. The bus goes on its lumbering way in such a circuitous route to the Marylebone Road that I ache from holding my ridiculous posture. I look at my watch: I have to get off and get a cab. There is one behind the bus. What luck. I spend several moments on the bus platform wondering whether I dare risk jumping off so near to the taxi. I realise, very slowly—because the ground is moving between the bus and the cab—that there is no way my brain can, or should, assess the gap.

The gynaecologist shows me sympathy and understanding of 'the terrible ordeal' I've been through, but I can only think with dread of the return journey. I cry and cry and cry. When she suggests an exploratory operation in three days' time, I agree at first and then I'm shocked at what I've done. I express doubts about blasting my poor head with yet more anaesthetic, and she suggests an epidural. I see, almost subliminally, that she is after another surgery fee. I get up and leave as politely as I can, saying I will think about it. That's a lie. I've thought. The answer's no. I don't go back.

'Ha, ha,' says Dr Lewith, the heavenly homeopath who treats me like a person. 'You're learning,' when I tell him of this.

But am I?

CHAPTER THIRTEEN

Midsummer Madness

My summer acting-school employers send the college driver to pick me up. A delightful chap, name of Albert, who, after hearing about my brainstorm, takes his eyes off the road, something I'm sure he never normally does, and turns to say, in the softest of Oxfordshire accents, 'Isn't this goin' to be a bit too much for you, this teachin'? Now, don't you go overdoin' it.'

I bubble inside and go to great lengths to explain that I don't know what I can do until I do it. It's not like an ordinary job, acting. I make myself stop because I'm getting het up and already feel alarmingly tired.

All I've done is pack my bags and close up the cottage, but at the back of my mind is the worry about sustaining a three-hour class. There's no preparation I can do for the class, it's a question of my responding in the moment to what the student offers, assessing where their shortcomings are vocally, physically and emotionally, and the way they manage the different demands of the structure of their piece of text. In the past it has slowly dawned on me that a two- to three-hour masterclass uses the same energy as the performance of a one-woman show. And I've got four lined up in a row. That's still only half a week's work in the theatre—four performances. Well, I'll certainly know where I am at the end of *that*.

My room overlooks the Tower of Balliol's frontage. Albert insists on carrying my bags up. We arrive at the door. It is locked. Disaster, I think. I cannot go down the stairs and come up again. 'Key!' says Albert, tut-tutting and tapping his head over our mutual forgetfulness. I berate myself for having forgotten that keys have to be picked up from the porter's lodge. I know this well, after all the summers I've taught here. Why does it matter that I forgot? Albert forgot too. Ah, but Albert hasn't had brain surgery.

When Albert goes smilingly to fetch the culprit key, Carolyn, *en route* to check on me with her motherly concern foremost, interrupts him in her eager, helpful way, and dashes off instead. I want to sink down into the coolness of the stone floor and sniff at the little spills of air coming through the gap between the door and the jamb. Albert says, 'You ought t' be sittin' down.'

'No, I'm—' I wave away his concern, trying to make light of it. He shakes his head dolefully in my direction. I try to visualise the coming evenings spent just drinking in the exquisite medievalness of what I will be able to see from the window of the room, along with the odd glass of Australian Cabernet Sauvignon, of course. If I can see this tantalising amount of the building from a cold and rather dark corridor it promises well. Carolyn returns triumphant with the key. 'Isn't she wonderful?' says Carolyn, nodding in my direction. She won't think that when the haywire brain is in the driving seat, I think.

Albert goes on slowly shaking his head.

When it comes to it, after teaching just the first day and getting uncharacteristically tetchy towards the end of the class, which shocked me—I'm a nice person: correction, I *used* to be a nice person—and made the younger-than-usual senior group uncomfortable, I come clean about my head, ask them not to take it personally and, if they can, to make allowances for me. This is greeted with a round of applause, which has me stifling a gulp into my handkerchief, struggling to get my breath back and leaving the class at the earliest permissible moment.

I can barely walk up the small flight of stairs to my room. It hurts to sit. It hurts to lie down. My whole body feels as if it has been skinned. Every nerve in every part feels as if it's exposed to the air. The dry air rakes across them. This is more than exhaustion. I have drawn on reserves, as I usually do when performing, pulling something extra out of the bag—what every actor does in rising to the occasion—but reserves, of course, are what I no longer have, if I ever did. Now, too, I have nothing to pull *with*. I am critically overdrawn. I am too tired to care what's out of the window. I am too tired to be. I just want oblivion. Oblivion will block out the rawness that's my body and the chattering, despairing nonsense that's my brain. I know now where I am all right, I am nowhere. Nowhere in Oxford with a bottle of Chilean Shiraz, seven months into my convalescence and three more classes to survive.

My day 'off' is spent getting to Warwick University and back. *En route* to Patricia, who's going to drive me, I stop at the cottage. There is a card there from the priest I wrote to in which he confirms what I'd suspected all along: the spirit of a recently deceased person *has* been causing me harm. Lines from the play we're working on at Balliol jump out at me. 'To whom should I complain? Did I tell this, who would believe me?' I am cautiously elated with relief. Then I rejoice. That takes energy. Then I have none. So then I worry. I'm like a bad Jewish joke. Things will get better now, I keep telling myself. I am joyful and thankful, but that too takes its toll. The honorary doctorate is duly bestowed. I think they gave it to me because they feel sorry for me. No, says the prof, who read the rather sparse eulogy, they didn't know I'd been ill. I wish my son could've made it. I know he's avoiding me. Wise fellow. I wish I could avoid me. All of the me's.

On my return to Oxford, crossing from one side of the quad to the other becomes a Herculean task. I am empty, however much tormented sleep or rest I have. My body is a vacant, throbbing, uninhabited space. An aching emptiness. I am just not in my body. Several colleagues, whom I haven't yet met, seem overjoyed to see me, envelop me in great hugs and then, holding my shoulders, step back and give me beaming, appraising smiles. Julian Glover says, 'My God, you did it! You damn well did it!' I can't think what he means at first and then, as I'm on the point of saying, 'I didn't do anything, it's luck, it's the French surgeons, it's—' a thought zaps across my consciousness: that *this* is where the extra joy that people show me comes from, some notion that I've beaten death, and if *I* have then *they* can too. But no one actually sits down with me and asks me about my head. Perhaps they are frightened that if they did I would tell them. My head is all I have.

As we stand in the cool of a huge tree Carolyn Sands, BADA's right hand and arm, passes. I'm still holding Julian's arm for support, and Carolyn, smiling her ever-benevolent smile, says to him, 'Isn't she wonderful?'

I say, 'I am stupid.'

Carolyn smiles. She is a lovely woman. Always ready to help with the dozens of things that can and do go wrong with students discovering the night life in Oxford and the genial licensing laws of Europe after the restrictions of the United States. She shakes her head admiringly and goes on her way.

'I mean it,' I say. I was always daft. Now I am stupid. 'I *am* stupid.' What I mean is, I am seriously stupid. I have pushed myself to the point of total collapse. I am frightened by how weak I feel. I am ashamed to admit even to myself the dread fact that can no longer be dodged. I feel worse now than I did when I came out of hospital in France. And, to top it all, I have a sore throat. I can't think of an area of my body that doesn't hurt. Perhaps my elbows. I am more than stupid. I am psychotically stupid.

In the car going back Albert says, 'You look

done in.'

'Yes, Albert,' I say, 'done in is what I am.'

Done in. Wiped out. Washed up.

And I did the doing.

I try some undoing. I cancel all my arrangements in London for the following week. I need rest. Rest and quiet. And help. I need a doctor. Quick.

CHAPTER FOURTEEN

At the Doctor's

I bike exhaustedly to the doctor's surgery through a grey, penetrating drizzle that suits my mood and feelings. It's slightly downhill on the way there. My spirits don't rise to the smallest flicker as the wind surges through my sweaty, matted hair on the slopes, as I know I simply won't be able to bike back. Just by the speed-limit sign on the outskirts of the town, shards of glass glint in my path. I swerve neatly to avoid them, am just beginning to feel smug that I did, when the bike starts to bump in a regular and jarring manner. I get off. The back wheel is utterly flat. Its tyre is sagging on to the Tarmac. I despair. I know a place that mends bikes in the town, but my eyes fill with tears nevertheless. I garner some intrigued looks. Middle-aged woman pushing a bike with a flat tyre, crying. Big deal.

By the time I get in to see Doc X I am a shaking, incoherent, inarticulate mess.

'So, how are you?'

I wish I felt smart-assed enough to say, 'So how are your powers of observation today?' But her mild question causes me to heave to keep the sobs down. Strings of snot run down my face as I wipe at it ineffectively with an already sodden, screwed-up Kleenex. I blurt out stuff I didn't even know I was harbouring. 'I can't sleep,' I bawl. I sound just like that child again. That pathetic, hopeless six-year-old. I was six when I found out my foster-mother wasn't my real mother. Except she was of course. She was the one who mothered me. The doc passes me some Kleenex from her box. This gesture brings fresh strangled retching. I *am* hopeless. What I mean is, I am without hope.

'I am hope-less.'

'Don't be silly.'

'I just need a hug, that's all.' I can't believe I'm coming out with such silliness.

'It's not just a hug, is it?' There's an implication of 'You and I know better.' 'You're depressed.'

It sounds like the accusation I'm sure it is. My mother suffered from depression. I inherited it. My foster-mother's biggest weapon was 'You'll turn out just like your mother.' So I couldn't. Because my mother

210

was bad. She had me at nineteen, and brought scandal on the old lady's house.

'Can't sleep,' I whine. 'Three pills a night.'

'Three sleeping tablets a night? You're only supposed—'

'I know—'

'Don't interrupt me—to take one.'

'I interrupt all the time.' A fresh crest billows up, which swoops and dips with me clinging to it.

'One tablet a night,' she repeats. I know this. I don't have dementia. I have insomnia.

I wish a middle-class wish. I wish I were with my private doctor in London. He treats me like a person. My private doctor knows he can trust me. He gives me repeat prescriptions in advance. But I can't afford to go and see him. He's in London. I hear my cleaning lady in my head saying of *her* treatment in the NHS, 'Its terrible being one of the herd.'

'Three?' She shakes her head. She is quietly aghast.

'Not all at once.' I manage a shred of self-defensiveness. 'I read, and then I read some more . . . and then I take another pill. My brain won't stop chattering.' My brain won't stop now.

'Look, look at you now. You're interrupting me again.'

'I know. I know. I'm sorry. I do it all the time. It's been worse since I've been ill. I snap at everyone. I hate the world and the world hates me.'

'No, the world doesn't hate you.' This is said gently. She smiles.

More heaving.

She stretches out her hand and strokes mine. I like this woman. She was kind when I first came to see her a couple of years ago. I bought her an Anita Shreve novel, *The Pilot's Wife*, that I thought was damn good escapism, well written too. God knows what in all this makes me howl, but howl I do.

'You are self-catastrophising.'

I want to laugh. This is a ridiculous word. It's so unwieldy. Perhaps it's new pop-psychology jargon. Perhaps it's American. Whatever it is, it's ugly. And, what's more, it's wrong.

'Well, you are an actress.'

Oh, that old onion. If I wasn't so low I'd gasp. Or send something flying. Preferably the nearest medic. 'I was—am, am a human being before I was an actor.' That seems to me like a lucid enough thing to say. I have a passion against people being labelled by what they do. 'Please don't label me. It's . . . it's like me saying you behave like a doctor . . . when you're . . . out . . . socially, all the time.' In fact, I'm rather pleased with the analogy. She looks at me quizzically.

'It's the symptoms of the cerebral haemorrhage . . . isn't it?' I hate that pleading tone in my voice. (Obsequious snake.) But I'm pleased I've come up with this thought. It has never struck me before. It feels right. A shard of light.

'You've been depressed before.' So it is *an* accusation. 'It's not just that, is it?' She says it in that professional, confidential you-and-I-both-know-otherwise-don't-we voice.

'I have a sore throat,' I say. But that wasn't what I meant at all.

She motions me to open my mouth. She holds my tongue down with a wooden spatula while my brain wheels, and I try to override the ever-increasing circles of thought in an attempt to hang on to what I was saying. What *was* I saying?

She puts the spatula down and gives me a long hard stare. I feel uncomfortable. I feel as if I have done something wrong. I thought this woman was my friend. I bought her a copy of one of my favourite books. Thoughts tumble and jumble.

'What is it that's changed your attitude to me?' Did I say that? At last. Space. Space. Space to speak the truth. Perhaps the symptoms are not all bad if they give me this freedom. I can think of quite a few people I would like to practise this on. There is silence in the room. Now it is her turn to look uncomfortable. I have no idea where the conversation is.

She wrote me a card to say she liked the book. It can't be that. My doctor in London chats to me about all sorts of things, where he's been on holiday, how his wife is, what plays he's seen lately—

'I realised I was treating you differently from my other patients. I was losing my grip.' I think she means she was developing a human relationship with me. Not just seeing me as a bundle of symptoms. A bumper bundle. However, I feel slapped down.

'In America,' where I feel loved and safe, I think, 'I—when I went—'

'You've been to America?' She sounds incredulous. I can't think why. People go to America all the time. Besides, now *she's* interrupting *me*.

I search around for something ordinary to say to stop her being so surprised. 'I was scared about what the plane would do to my head. It did feel . . . odd at first. I felt things shifting. Inside my head. When it first took off things moved—I *can* feel my brain . . .' I'm not making sense.

'But the surgeon in France said I could fly back from Paris . . .'

'America?'

'Yes.' I thought we were talking about Paris. 'They're my friends. I love them. They love me.' Thin ice. I know I am starting to wobble. But, I think, I could never have said that I knew people loved me . . . BC. The back of my throat is stinging with more than the soreness. 'They wanted to look after me.' With this, my last bastion is washed away. 'I had to go,' I

214

snivel. 'The university paid for the air fare. I did a masterclass.'

'You've been teaching?'

'Yes, just one class. It was fine. Well, no, it wasn't. I wasn't present.' That's an acting term. She won't understand that. 'I mean, I didn't know. Where I was . . . I felt vague . . . dizzy . . . I've done—'

'Stop talking. Just stop talking—'

'—four now here. Not here. In Oxford.' This is all becoming a terrible scramble in my head. I make a desperate attempt to straighten it all out. 'I teach in Oxford every year—'

'Stop interrupting me. You keep interrupting me.' She types something into her computer. She's right. So I do.

'I had to find out how much I could do.'

'How much?'

Momentarily I lose the thread. I can't live on the money coming in. 'I have to sell my house to get the money—'

'Just a minute.' She clicks some more keys on her computer. Doesn't she know how hard it is for me to wait? How hard it is for me to hang on to what I was saying? She's a doctor, she should know.

'What were you saying?'

What *was* I saying? I now have an absolutely vacant mind. I have no idea why I am here or what I came for. A fresh phalanx of teardrops lines up and spills over the back of my hand.

'You're depressed. You're clinically depressed,'

215

she says again. I have no idea what clinical is either. I don't know what I know and what I don't know.

'Do you want to talk to someone, a psychiatrist?'

I nod. The prospect of having some help with all of this brings a vast wave of relief.

'She's private. You can't see her on the National Health. Can you afford it?'

'No.'

'And your son, have you seen him?'

I can't speak. I shake my head.

'And Ann?'

I shake my head more vigorously

'You *are* in a state.' Again I hear the accusation. So it *is* all my fault.

'I don't feel well.' This comes out in a childlike wail.

'I don't think it's the brain operation. I think it's everything else in your life.'

Oh, thanks for the help, my life's a mess, she thinks. I think so too. Then I feel a sting of unfairness. A flicker of rage starts to uncurl quietly, deep inside. I start again: 'I had to go to America so they c-c-c-c-could look after me. I have to g-g-g-go to London to sell the house.'

It doesn't come out quite like the strong and direct statement I'd ordered. It sounds pathetic. I feel pathetic. I give up. So does she.

'There's a room up the corridor where you can sit. I have to get on.' She gives up too. I feel again as if I've been slapped.

There was something else. I try to stand up. My hands are shaking. Even if the bike shop's fixed the bike, I'll never manage to cycle back now. I'll have to cadge a lift in the square. What was it I must remember? I must remember. Oh, yes.

'Sickness certificate? I need—runs out tomorrow.'

There's a pause.

'No.'

'What?'

'You can work.'

'I can't do eight shows a week,' I blurt. I couldn't do one. I couldn't even *get* to the theatre. I am flabbergasted. My chest feels tight. It is hard to breathe. 'I couldn't—'

'I am saying that you *could* work. Not necessarily *your* work. You go to London. You've been to America—'

'Yes, but—' The injustice of it has me reeling. I cannot believe what I have heard. It is not believable.

'Don't interrupt. You cycled here.'

I think, So it would be better if I didn't try. Would it be better if I sat all day on a sofa saying 'I can't. I can't do anything'? I have never found it easy to say I can't. In the silence of the room someone says, 'I can't.' I flinch. She stares at me. 'I c-c-c-can't always get a lift in . . . to shop, here in . . . a car. I have to be independent.' Were there too many ins in that sentence? What was it that just shocked me?

'Did you go to see the brain surgeon I recommended?'

'No.' Again I am in the wrong. I am upset. Why am I upset? 'Work,' I repeat dumbly.

'Yes.'

'As a . . . a . . . receptionist?' It's the only job I can think of where I could sit down all day. A job that needs no skills.

'Well . . . Yes.'

All the voices in my head clamour for precedence: 'But I've been an actor for thirty-five years'; 'I've never done another job'; 'This is the first time in my life I've claimed sickness benefit.'

The printer goes on chugging out the prescriptions.

'A receptionist?' I need to check that I heard right. She gives me nothing for my sore throat. More sleeping tablets for my dreadful nights and anti-depressants for my state. I am grateful for the sleeping tablets even if they don't work. For me, anti-depressants have always been synonymous with failure. My mother was on them for most of her life.

'A receptionist,' I say quietly to myself.

'Yes,' she says, handing me the prescriptions.

I do not know how I'm going to manage on fifty pounds less coming in each week. But I do know that if what she has just said is sanity, then now there is no doubt I am insane.

218

CHAPTER FIFTEEN

BASIC Help

My home won't sell. The dream flat has gone to someone who isn't waiting to sell and has ready cash to buy. All my hopes are dashed. Darleney makes light of it, brushes it aside and comes up to spend a few days with me in the country. The sun shines, I am not alone, we go for walks in a countryside that is brimming with life and I feel truly and wholeheartedly glad to be part of it. I have to stop several times on the hill to catch my breath and wonder where the energy is going to come from to make it to the top, while she strides ahead easily. I choose not to note it too much.

I see an advert for a walk in the Andes to raise money for Dr Barnardo's. After several exasperating phone calls, each one marginally more frustrating than the last as I have to go through the rigmarole of repeating the details each time, I finally locate the PR officer who's in charge of publicity for the expedition and, trying to shed the build-up of irritation, explain that I'm the ideal candidate. My mother was a Barnardo's girl before she was fostered; she's not long been dead—I mutter something about expiation; I've just survived brain surgery; I'm crazy about the Andes, always wanted to go to Peru; and I love walking. It seems like a marriage made in heaven. Darleney is very enthusiastic and supportive. So is the girl at Barnardo's. We plan to talk in a couple of months' time. It shocks me that I'm able now to think in months not days, but I feel elated that at last I am going to do something positive with all this . . . all this Time Off.

In a frantic but sustained bout of telephoning, in which the Dr Barnardo's call is relatively minor, I finally locate a support group. I get more sympathy and understanding from a Sandra Buckley who mans a telephone helpline called BASIC for people with brain or spinal injuries than I have had from the medical profession in nine months. In our short conversation I find out that she herself suffered a cerebral haemorrhage some eleven years ago. Immediately everything she says has a forceful quality and clarity that zings down the line and forges a direct connection with me.

'I'm much harder on myself now than I was before.'

'I'm more selfish now.'

'It seems as if the exhaustion will never end.'

'It's taken over my life.'

I do not know which of us is speaking.

The next support group meeting is, as it happens, at Mr Y's hospital. I am appalled that he seemed not to know of it. But, as I am to learn many times in the coming months, the medical profession has clear demarcation lines. His surgeon's job ends at the operating-theatre door.

The meeting coincides with my next visit to London to restart the flat hunt. I try to learn more poems on the train. I don't realise that I am mouthing the words until I catch the look of a man sitting opposite. As I lock eyes with him, I have an overpowering desire to stick my tongue out. It is so strong an urge and it feels so right that I have to force myself to look down at the text for fear of carrying it out. And it's not a teasing-tip-of-the-tongue-you-cheeky-thing, but a sod-you-who-the-fuck-do-you-think-you're-looking-at?

I shock myself.

Apart from the support group meeting—which I am really looking forward to—I plan to see a wise old woman, the WOW, in London to make my visit more of a pleasure than just a disheartening estate-agent-bound chore. I have been in the habit of visiting her for some years now, but I haven't seen her since I fell ill. She always gets up and walks down the three flights of stairs each time the doorbell rings and walks back up without so much as a puff or a pant. I hold on to the banister and count off each step as I climb, never having been aware before of just how numerous they are.

It is, as always, a delight to see her. She

221

exudes serenity. Her movements are gentle and controlled. She is utterly, at every moment, in touch with herself. Being a Jungian therapist could well have something to do with it. She must be well into her eighties, but her eyes have the brightness and alertness of the spirit of a young girl. The large, light room with its ceiling-to-floor windows and prospering green plants is dense with peace. I drink it in. In this room my head slows down. The chatter is still there but somehow I can ignore it, rise above it. Or duck beneath it. There is something about her presence that solicits only what is important from me. I seem to be able, under her concentrated gaze, to sift through the clamour and get to the essence of things. She closes the door softly behind her and walks to the fireplace where she stoops to pick up a large candle which she lights.

She then turns to me and says, smiling, 'You have a new life. Happy New-Birth day.' Something in me, thanks to her, at last rejoices. We talk of the night sea voyage, the journey to individuation. My son. How I didn't want them to cut my nails off because of sticking Callas's on top. How mad they must have thought me. She laughs. How I tricked Dr Vinikoff into thinking my hair had turned white overnight with the shock. My son. How important it has been for me to break the cycle of bad mothering. To lay that ghost. And the ghost that is now laid. How anger can get broken off. In girls most of all. How angry my son is. How angry the new me is—the new mes are. We laugh. The friends that anger has cost me. 'She wiped your bottom. You were her baby. She didn't like it when the teenager left home.' It all makes sense. She tells me how her thirty-four-year-old son now puts her on his knee and says, 'Mama, it's all your fault.' We laugh.

I leave her some hour later, light of heart and head, smiling like a lunatic at everyone I pass on the street. I feel washed clean, new and carefree, at least until I get to the Northern Line. Its screeches make me wince. No one else in the carriage seems to notice. I can't think why they don't, it's unbearably loud, but I am so suffused with calm it hardly matters. As a nightcap, I knit a bit more scarf, drink some good South Eastern Australian Cabernet, and sleep and sleep.

The support group is a shambles. Apart from no one at the hospital knowing if, or where, it is taking place, there are precious few people about to ask: the reception area seems deserted and it is only seven in the evening. When it finally convenes, there are twelve to fifteen people, mostly women, and everyone talks at once. All the time. There is someone in a uniform too, but she makes no effort to introduce herself, to co-ordinate the group or explain why or what the purpose of the meeting is.

The girl sitting beside me, who is astonishingly only in her early thirties, had such a crashing pain in her head in a nightclub in Majorca that she thought someone had spiked her drink. Only hours later did she and her friends grasp that there was something wrong with her head. She tells the whole story with an abrasive, self-defensive, querulous air that irks me, but that I have to admit I recognise.

A suntanned, late middle-aged couple sit opposite me. She, resplendent in many golden necklaces and rings, and her husband of many years, who is patently devoted to her and who has only marginally fewer decorations, express the situation they have been through in the matter-of-fact tones of the much-experienced. He has stuck by her through inexplicable mood swings, irrational tears and fretful irritability. I wonder if she knows how lucky she is to have him. Only seconds later she takes his hand and they are lost to us while they smile deeply at each other. I realise that they are not here because they have a problem to solve. They have solved it by living through it. 'Oh, it'll take two or three years just to get over the exhaustion of it,' she says to the group at large. 'I mean, I still have days that I don't know how to get through,' she nods at him in a knowing manner, 'and I've never gone back to work full-time. He's done extra to make up for it. You've had to work extra, haven't you, haven't you?' Now it's his turn to nod.

Two to three years of this. I'm dumbstruck. I can't bear to think of it. The longer I'm in this damned convalescence the more the end of it seems to recede.

To the right of the young girl taken ill on holiday is another young woman. She is evidently distraught. She fidgets in her chair and absentmindedly pats her hair, presumably over the place where the scar is. She has a young child whom she has, yet again, she says, dumped on her husband while she talks, yet again about her bloody brain haemorrhage. 'I can't talk about anything else,' she says. 'I couldn't care less about the baby—well, I could, really. But I can't get over what has happened to me. This brain haemorrhage has taken over my whole life. It's all I talk about. I bore my husband, I bore my friends.'

I want to stand up and shout, 'Me too. Me too.' I am so relieved I want to hug her. I am so grateful that she has described her obsession in such a way that it almost assuages me about my own. This does a bit to alleviate the doom-laden timespan of two, three years.

To her right is an elderly lady with a trim grey bob. 'Well, I've got two,' she says, somewhat proudly.

My ears prick up at this.

'Two what?' someone asks.

225

'Aneurysms,' she says, somewhat crossly, as if the questioner should know better.

She then goes on to explain in minute detail the step-by-step clipping of the first. The procedure doesn't resemble what I've been through, but my attention is hooked. I lose track of what she said, and then what the doctor had said, and then what she replied to what the doctor had said, but I salvage enough of the goings-on to be able to ask my pressing question when she stops long enough to draw breath.

'When did this happen?' I enquire rather timidly, my voice sounding so unlike my own that I sound apologetic for speaking out at all. This has just the opposite effect of the one I had desired and everyone looks at me. 'I've got a second one too,' I mumble.

'Nineteen years ago,' she retorts triumphantly. Nineteen years and she's still talking about it! I am too appalled to despair. I want to scream with derision.

'Don't you think the chances of it bursting now are slightly remote?' I say icily, irritated and tired beyond measure. There is an uncomfortable lull in the room. In the next general outburst of chatter, thinking it an irony that here, of all places, I can't bear the noise, I get up disappointed, exhausted, and leave. I feel very spare.

I finish the red scarf, cast around in my mind who to give it to, and worry about what to do next to keep my hands occupied while I sit and sit. I shouldn't have mentioned the stream of blood the scarf reminds me of, but at least I withhold from describing the flecks in the wool as bits of brain. Nevertheless the man friend I offer it to declines it politely, explaining that he doesn't much want my pain wrapped round his neck. There's nothing for it, come winter, but to wrap it round my own.

I arrive back from London, nerves jangled, no new flats to ruminate on, feeling grimy and uncomfortable just in time for the pre-arranged visit by a dear friend, Ray, and his sister. I hardly know the sister at all, but I snap at her when she compares what she thinks I have achieved in my life with what she thinks she hasn't in hers. And the award for bad timing goes to . . . But she wasn't to know, poor girl. I am unaccountably cross. I can't believe that I am so angry with someone I barely know, except that I read her self-pity clearly, loathe it and verbally smack her down for it. Ray doesn't try to defend her or placate me. I go on to explain the importance of the many unnoticed little acts of kindness she must have performed throughout her life in her job at the office till I sound like Patience Strong.
 I ignore that I also sound like a self-

righteous prig. I go on and on, making matters worse. I can't help it. I am compelled to speak the truth and I can't stop talking. The uncomfortable atmosphere with which I, singlehandedly, have soiled the afternoon pervades the cottage like an unpleasant smell. Later, over tea, which does nothing to dispel the gloom, I tell Ray, an experienced walker, of my plan to go walking in the Andes. Quietly and deferentially he suggests I sleep outside in the cottage garden for four or five nights in a row to get used to the roughness and the low temperature I will encounter sleeping outside in Peru. I am crestfallen and duly abashed. 'You have to be fighting fit to take on something like that,' he says gently. Fighting fit. Hm. I've cornered the fighting bit.

Better stick to the poems.

The day of the poetry recital I attend a farewell celebration for an actor friend at the Swan theatre in the afternoon and have to leave early to rehearse the recital at the Shakespeare Centre. I feel as if I am in a time warp as I run through the streets of Stratford clutching my recital clothes in a hanging bag. I have always been running through the streets of Stratford on some sort of time-loop because now, too, I am late for rehearsal. It only strikes me as I slow down, because my head begins to spin, that the people whose feet I picked my

228

way past in the auditorium, many of whom I knew, may well have supposed I was leaving early because I was unwell. That worries me, until I am caught up in the sheer joy of working with Paul and Norman, laughing at each other's silliness, as actors do when there is no director around, and focusing blessedly on the poetry, most of which I feel reasonably confident about as I have learned by heart so many of the poems.

It is just as well that I have: during the actual performance I am so exhilarated to be standing on a stage again—albeit in a lecture hall and not a theatre—and so comforted by the companionship of Paul and Norman at either side of me that the adrenaline threatens to lift me off my feet. I feel as if I am all air. I am completely unconnected to the ground. I am just a voice and a head. I make myself concentrate for every second of the evening as I am terrified of what will happen if I don't. Certain of the poems that I have to read, which deal with death, have an inexplicable edge and sharpness that doesn't come from me, I realise, but are informed by the experience I have been through. Several friends from the theatre club in Bristol comment on this later, diminishing the fear that it was my particular delusion. The overriding impression that I have of the entire evening, as Darleney drives me back through the dark country lanes in her wonky little car, is how much I love my job. How unspeakably glad I am to have found this love again for a job that I toyed with giving up before I was ill. The theatre. How my stepfather Lapotaire and real mother tried to prevent me doing it. How stubborn and determined I was. How I love the theatre. This is a huge solace. I feel enormous inside, full of hope and elated with joy. Supper and several glasses of wine do little to ground me. Darleney listens patiently and kindly to my excited recollections of the evening. She knows, too, what an important and significant watershed this recital has been for me. I have to recall more soberly, though, that the exultation of the evening and the adrenaline-flow in my weak system were so enormous that it would have taken little at any point to knock me flat.

And knocked flat is what I am, for days on end, with crippling headaches that painkillers barely touch. I hug an ice-pack to my head while I lie in bed, tie it round my neck with a tea-towel, shove it down my T-shirt when I lie on the floor, desperate for the small of my back, which aches as if it has been kicked, to be relieved by the smoothness and the coolness of the flagstones that I can sense under the thin carpet. But relief is not to be had. In fact, true to form, I am my own worst enemy. I misjudge the low beam in the kitchen and walk smack into it. I want to laugh at the irony of hitting my head, but I yelp out loud, like the child who seems to accompany me most of the time and gets very vocal in moments of particular direness. I rub my head while my eyes smart and sting. I rub it and rub it just like my foster-mother did when I was little.

Darleney is preparing to go home to Australia for several months to deal with family business and take in the Olympic Games, so any flat-hunting will have to be accomplished alone, and without, too, that particularly appreciated kindness: her meeting me at the station.

So I will be back to coping single-handed with the monster that I have become and the animals in the zoo that is London.

CHAPTER SIXTEEN

Time Off?

Most of the people I know in the village are away on holiday, so as the head pain reluctantly abates, I try to divide my time between slowly clearing the pile of mail that builds up when I add the latest load from London to the already substantial pile in the cottage, and lounging in the garden. I had envisaged weeks and weeks stretching ahead of days in the sun, but the weather has other ideas. Meteorology doesn't know that this is the first summer I've had off in thirty-five years. I feel thoroughly cheated of the sun. I take up knitting again, with a very sullen will. Except that this time it's a bright periwinkle-blue scarf for my dear eighty-seven-year-old friend Floy, who has eyes of that colour and a mass of white hair. In a moment of tiredness I had been rather short with her. I love this old lady. We gossip about actors and the theatre, catch up on all the scandal, have sherry over ice cubes—a particular Australian treat of hers—and when I stop going on and on about my bloody brain for long enough we have lots of laughs. That I should have been bad-tempered with her of all people . . . She had mentioned that someone in the village shop had remarked on my behaviour, and she had said, 'She has been *very* ill, you know.' That old paranoia had me in its spell and I snapped at her. It preyed on my mind all one night. It grew into a huge problem until I could apologise to her. She dismissed it with a 'Darling, if you can't get cross with me . . .? I love you.' I realised that she did love me. I realise, too, that I have lost my sense of proportion. I wonder in which area of the brain a sense of proportion resides—obviously not far from the sense of humour, as that's gone on the slide too. There are so few people I feel at ease with now. I was made aware, by this incident in particular, that it's no good being looked after by people, however kind, who don't love you. Only love helps to ride out the hard bits.

Among the mail I find a letter from the National Hospital for Neurology informing me of an appointment. This makes me totally paranoid. Who arranged this appointment? How did they know my address? Why wasn't I told about it? What's it for? I suspect it might be the private insurance company checking on my validity to go on drawing the small pension. This, of course, is a preposterous idea, but I guess it is born from my feelings of guilt about being paid to do nothing. Or, rather, considering the pain and frailty that is the accompaniment to this time off, that I am receiving money I am not able to work for. Conveniently forgetting, of course, that I have been paying into this fund for years and years.

I spend an age on the telephone trying to get through to the hospital switchboard. When I do get through it's an automatic voice, none of whose options fits my request. I scream abuse down the phone. By the time I manage to speak to a person I am so overwrought that I am barely polite. I end up none the wiser about the appointment with a shadow of paranoia that doggedly remains.

Urged on by the general disappearance of the village on holiday and the idea of doing something constructive with all this so-called free time, in one morning I sign myself up for a Quaker retreat at their centre in Birmingham, decide to attend the Guild of Pastoral Psychology's annual conference in Oxford—I have been a member for some years—and then, really in the swing with the holiday notion, beg to borrow a friend's small flat in the old town of Ibiza. I brush aside any worries that I might, with reason, entertain about being felled by similar dastardly head pains in foreign places.

I notice, tucked discreetly away in the corner of the dashboard of a friend's car, a toy lion cub. It is very lifelike. It has a cold nose (plastic) and beseeching eyes (glass). It is exactly like the one in the dream. I am not, nor ever have been, a furry toy person. In fact, I never had any furry toys as a kid. My big love was a rag doll called Josephine. But this cub is so lifelike, and so like the one in the dream, that I have to have it. Or one very like it. I pick it up, stroke it and talk to it. My friend makes a kind of snuffling noise. I'm not sure whether it's a snuffle of approval or embarrassment. I suspect the latter.

I spend a long time on the phone the following day—I have never used the phone so much as I do these days. Well, I can socialise without facing the terrors of the times— crowds, mobile phones, bass beats—that's if

I'm not bursting a blood vessel in exasperation with the other end of the line, of course. I track down the World Wildlife Fund HQ. The lion cub is out of stock. I simply won't be told no. The young woman at the other end of the line is party to this brain-crazed obsession, which is probably why she makes that extra effort. Eventually she finds two sitting on someone's desk. I buy them both. When they arrive I am relieved I live alone as the six-year-old is given free rein. The kitchen reverberates with words of welcome and giggles of delight. I despatch the second cub to my unsuspecting son and, with much delight, put mine to guard my sleep and doze off with my fingers deep in its fur. A fifty-five-year-old six-year-old.

The four days of the Quaker retreat (one of them spent in silence) help me find a small pool of blessed quiet inside myself at last. But my body doesn't much like the discipline of sitting still three times a day for half an hour each time. My ankles swell up alarmingly. I look down at them and see the legs and feet of my foster-mother, who was in her mid-nineties when she died. I feel so unwell I have to miss all of one afternoon's classes while I rest in my little monk-like cell.

It seems such an irony that here, in the centre of an institution founded on silence, the chairs in the refectory make such loud scraping noises on the wooden floor that I flinch. If I turn down my hearing-aid I can't hear what people are saying; if it's up, I want to scream at the noise as it scrapes the inside of my head. A real Catch 22 except it feels 44. I so relish the meals that are taken in silence—apart from the din of the chairs, of course—the welcome relief of not having to communicate with anyone, not having to make an effort to get to know people. Just eating delicious food that I haven't had to shop for and prepare myself, in the presence of other people for whom silence is essential. I am so grateful for this place I want to weep into my homemade soup. Instead I weep all over a dear lady, who is an Elder; she catches me as I'm coming down the stairs after my afternoon off. Her kindness and concern for me are so evident that the tears flow all too easily. She takes me to her room and tells me gently of her struggles to survive when her husband died and she had to move to a smaller flat. How utterly alone she felt. She tells me, even more gently, that my convalescence may take a lot longer than I think. She is so placid and composed that for the first time in seven months I don't find the idea at all alarming. 'Disencumber' is her favourite word. Disencumber! Yes! I see it all clearly. I will sell everything in the house, sell the house and live on the money. Simple. Oh, and I'll learn the piano too. I've always wanted to play the piano.

236

I leave the retreat refreshed and renewed, apart from backache incurred by the wafer-thin sponge mattress on the bed. I have to get the back sorted before my next trip to the hellhole that is London, which is two days away. Good osteopath, back sorted, simple.

Of course, it is simple while moving remains just an idea. Simple, until I see all the little belongings I have at home that tug at my memory again. It's salutary, too, that I remember, so far, no one has wanted to buy my house. It's almost as if the house doesn't want to be sold. Darlene, whose tolerance of such occult nonsense is non-existent, reminds me in her parting shot that disencumbering is all very well but I will need somewhere in London for when I work. Work. Oh, yes. Uncannily the agent rings with an interview for a TV job. I combine flat-looking with the interview.

The job is four days of filming with two days off in the middle. Ideal. I won't be working for more than a couple of hours on each of those days. A small part. It's being directed by a young man I knew when he was an assistant director at the RSC. He apologises for the size of the role but thinks it will help me get my toes back in the water. The only significant characteristic of this woman is that she's a retired ballet dancer who can still put her hands flat on the floor when bending over. I walk into the interview and put my hands flat on the floor. It's bravado on my part. To hide the scared woman I am. Scared at being back in the real world. Scared at facing how much this illness has cost me in terms of what other people think I can do. Scared of knowing that I don't know what I can't do. Plain scared. After much joking and renewing of acquaintances they offer me the role and I leave. The sun is bright, my spirits are high. The job will pay for the holiday in Ibiza. Perfect. I have almost two months to get really strong before the filming. Two months. That's an age, I pretend to myself.

I see the second dream flat only doors away from the first, and put in a ridiculously high offer for it.

The bravado costs dear. It costs a pounding headache that worsens over several days and takes several visits to the London osteopath to clear. It's the first time I've seen him since my brain burst. He's a tall, gentle, caring man. He scoops me up with such a hug when he sees me, flushing pink with pleasure. He's Yugoslavian, so he knows about pain.

'My God,' he says, 'how good it is to see you.' We both laugh and giggle. Then he holds me at arm's length, observes me and says, in a quiet, sober tone, 'Do you *know* how lucky you are? Do you *know*?'

Equally seriously, I say, 'Oh, yes.'

The train coming back is cool The sun is pounding down outside, but for once the train is on time *and* the air-conditioning is working. Life can't get any better. The deep cream-coloured wheatfields whiz past. I don't want the flickering to irritate my newly cool, calm head, so I roll up my jacket and gingerly place my head on it, then settle between the edge of the backrest and the window. I feel becalmed inside. It is an odd, unusual feeling. I stay with it a few more moments before it dawns on me that I am feeling well. Well, not exactly well, as in bursting with health and vigour, but equable. Yes, that's it. Equable. Suddenly horizons are opening, anything seems possible. I have hope once more. Then I realise that the anti-depressants must be working at last. My mother's ghost judders into life for a few seconds. She made four suicide attempts even on happy pills. I dismiss the image. I am not nor ever have been my mother. Well . . . and then again . . .

The brain bash has given me a small but real sense of self-worth. I manage the unmanageable and sleep for a few minutes on a train.

Days later, in this state of benevolence, I am picking raspberries to make jam at the fruit farm at the top of the hill. I don't eat raspberry jam, but it's something to do, something to make. I am alone in the rows and rows of raspberry canes. The sun isn't as fierce as it was, and there is a gentle breeze that ruffles the green leaves into showing their silver undersides. I am overcome with the peace of it all. The sun is warm on my back. I feel it easing my very bones. What I think is a skylark offers up its full-throated song nearby. I stand still for a few seconds, close my eyes and offer up mine.

The room I am given at the Oxford college where the Guild of Pastoral Psychology conference is, does its share to extend this blessed period of peace. It has a curved bay window that overlooks the river; in fact, the half of the building that I am in extends over the water. It is a delight. I think of Mariana in the moated grange. I watch the shadows of the overhanging trees dapple the water. Ducks and moorhens scuttle about in the reeds at the water's edge. A swan is asleep with its head tucked into its wing as I unpack and settle in. I spend a long time staring out of the window, until I catch myself. I feel momentarily guilty as if I should be getting on with something. Then I remember that there is nothing to be getting on with except getting better, and that seems to be beyond my control. At long last I feel as if I am now well enough, paradoxically, to be able to enjoy being unwell. I rest every afternoon, which I have been half-hearted about doing when I am alone, largely because it reminds me that I'm ill. Also, by the time my body is screaming with tiredness, I know that twenty minutes on the floor in the Alexander technique posture won't be anywhere near enough to unwind all the winding up I've done. It takes sometimes an hour for me even to begin to relax. Whereas here, after two morning sessions and a coffee break, I badly need to get away from people, chatting, movement and laughter.

Appropriately, the subject of the conference this year is Death and Rebirth. 'Not a load of laughs there, then,' says Peter, who drives me yet again to the station. I wonder if—but I know I will bump into the doctor friend to whom I was very close for several years and who introduced me to the GOPP. We went frequently to lectures together and to hear the Reverend Dr Martin Israel preach his luminous sermons. Later, when I collapsed with exhaustion having got my son to university, she hospitalised me with what she called post-viral syndrome. She did me no favours calling it that. I got labelled when I returned to work as having had a nervous breakdown, when in fact what I had, have, is ME. She is the first person I bump into. Out of the two hundred or so people here, her room is next door to mine.

There are lectures given by a London rabbi, a doctor who manages a cancer hospice in Dublin, an elderly Canadian therapist, who

241

frankly reveals the problems he has in accepting the ageing process, and a learned astrologer who is also an accomplished musician. We meet every morning before the day begins for a quiet time, which is non-denominational.

It is during these sessions that I become aware of a man who says his prayers louder and slower than anyone else in the room. The voice has a condescending, patronising tone, and the vowels are drawn out in it, as if it is aping someone of so-called better breeding. It grates on my ear and offends my sensibilities no end. It is an odd quirk, this pretentious voice, especially in this company of priests, psychologists and therapists, people who, I assume, have more than a smattering of self-knowledge. When the owner of the voice stands up in the main lecture hall as the chair of an afternoon session, I see that it belongs to a bull-headed man with uneven tombstone-like teeth, a mouth of large rubbery pink lips that is awash with saliva, huge podgy hands with fat fingers that are only marginally less disturbing than the fat, hairy toes that poke out from his sandals, replete with ridged yellow talons ingrained with dirt. I can barely restrain myself, so full of disgust I am. I want to decry him as ugly, fat, repulsive, condescending, patronising—I cannot understand how anyone in the room can tolerate looking at him, let alone listening to his hideously phoney voice. I want to shout him down and beg the room to get up and go. I am bursting with outrage and dislike.

Later I learn that he is an analyst, am chastened to hear that he is particularly good at treating patients who are borderline insane. I also learn that the violence of my reaction, a state that stays with me for the rest of the last day and half of the conference, means that I am still, worryingly, far from well. But at least I know what my shadow looks like.

I do need that holiday. But there are two small hurdles to be faced before I can escape like everyone else: the TV job read-through and, at my own insistence, the EEG test. Well, I'm familiar with the work set-up, I think, so that'll be a doddle, but the EEG is worrying. What will it show? The second aneurysm emits little bleeps of terror whenever I allow my attention to scan it. I cannot conceive of enduring for a second time the journey I've come on this far.

After the chaos of the support group, the EEG test, which takes place in the same hospital, is so mundane that it is something of an anticlimax. A woman in a white coat places electrodes all over my head, and goes to great lengths to assure me that there will be no pain. I want to snap back in the face of her placidity that of course I know there will be no pain,

243

I've only had brain surgery, I'm not a congenital idiot. Then I remember that I don't know the difference between congenital and hereditary.

I am cross with myself for being so tired. All I've done is travel to London and about ten stops on the tube. I try to enlist her understanding of how tired and confused I am by explaining all the conflicting views I've had from the different medics with whom I've come into contact over the last eight months. Each of my horror stories is met with a non-committal 'Oh,' till I realise I'm talking to a woman who operates a machine and has no medical training opinions whatsoever.

A variety of lights of varying rhythms and brightness are shone into my eyes. It feels a bit like driving down the wrong lane of the motorway and having all the lights of the oncoming vehicles alarmingly near. It's more irritating than dramatic. It leads me to wondering, after a particularly sustained bout of short sharp flashes, what would happen if these lights triggered a fit. Well, I'm in a hospital, I muse, presumably they could handle it. Although these days, with the NHS, you never know. Then I wonder out loud what this test is going to be compared *with*? 'There is no EEG test of my brain *before* I was ill,' I say, in combative mood. 'Supposing,' I say, 'van Gogh, a teenager with Down's syndrome and I all had EEG tests, who's to say which is normal?' There is not a sound in the room. 'Or is it just to ascertain whether there is a potential for epilepsy?' I relish such comparisons, especially with the scientific fraternity, who can only function if everything is reduced to measurable quotas. But again I get no response. The test, all of twenty minutes or so, ends abruptly, and I wait for her to look at whatever she's just done and tell me the worst. Instead she says that the radiologist will inform Mr Y how to read it. Oh, no. Mr Y is not reading any more to do with me, I think, and I triumph inwardly as I remember the fast-approaching appointment with the National Hospital of Neurology. As she helps me on with my jacket, I realise that I have done more supposing in her small room in a short space of time than she probably thinks fit or needful. I want to put my head on her shoulder and say, 'I'm sorry.' I want her to offer me a cup of tea. I want for us to sit down and have a chat. I want anything, as long as I don't have to face the traffic and the noise and the crowds. She says, in a rather prim manner as she straightens my lapel, 'Now, you take good care of yourself and don't go overdoing it.' I want to push her out of my way.

I stagger about the kitchen trying to cook dinner for friends Stephen, Paul and Cherry. Even though I am clumsy when I'm normally deft and it all seems to go so slowly I do have something to celebrate. I am going back to work tomorrow. I raise a glass and thank them for having been such good friends. 'God knows,' says Stephen, 'it hasn't been easy.'

Sometimes I have the luxury of a driver when working on a film or a TV programme, but this role is so small that for the read-through at least I have to take the tube to Uxbridge and they will drive me from there. The read-through takes place in a large room in the film studios. Forty or so people, from every department of the film—makeup, wardrobe, camera crew, lighting, production office, and actors—assemble round a very long table. The director displays his prodigious memory of everyone he's employed to help him do this job; introduces us all to each other, and then we read the script. There are several faces round the table that I know well, and many warm, cheery greetings before we settle down. I feel slightly dazed by the number of people in the room, bewildered by the level of chatter and laughter, and wish I had made a decision about whether to mention my illness or not before I got here. I feel my anxiety grow. I see it all before me as if it is happening at a great distance from me. I feel no part of it. The actors are swapping stories about the last job they did. I listen to them. I am unable to join

246

in. I stand shakily not knowing what to do or where to look. With each greeting, I feel another wispy shred of strength leeched out of me. Some hugs threaten to topple me, I am so unsure of my feet or the ground.

As the room quietens for the reading, a small snake of terror uncurls itself from the pit of my stomach and makes its way slowly up my throat. Supposing I slur my words? I often do now, when I'm tired. I notice it if I talk on the phone late at night, or when I'm upset. Supposing I can't keep up? Supposing I lose my place? The read-through begins. This being a detective story it has a complex plot. I didn't understand it when I read it to myself at home and I don't understand it now. I've never cared about who-dun-it or where-they-dun-it or why. But it is imperative for me to understand this now, or I will know that my brain is stopping me understanding. A dear colleague, Mick F, opposite, whom I've worked with before, leans across the table in a lull of chatter, and says, 'Don't fret. Nobody understands these things.' But I know he's just being nice. I know he knows I've been ill, though he hasn't acknowledged it. So fret I do. There is so much I don't understand, but I daren't voice all my stupid questions, or they'll know just exactly how brain-damaged I am. I am wearing myself down.

Later, during the coffee break, when we've all scattered out into the cooling shade of the trees, the director wanders over to me to discuss what he thinks my character should wear. I am astonished at the vehemence with which I contradict him. I hadn't planned this. I hadn't really thought much about it at all. I know how inappropriate my reaction is from the look of surprise I see on his face, and on the face of the other person in our small group. I feel very hot. I wish I was sitting down again. I wish almost anything, other than being in this situation. Even the money doesn't seem to matter right now.

I say something, to prove to myself that I am connected to what's going on. I realise I must have interrupted the director rather abruptly by the sharp and insistent way he responds. I am making bad worse. I don't really know why. I try to explain to myself, as much as to them, that I do steamroller people since I've been ill. Then my own world closes in on me again as I wonder if I always did. Is this burning urgency to speak the instant I think of something a symptom of 'the illness' or a fixture? A part of me that either I chose not to see before or a part that was somehow broken off that now makes up the whole? As if the illness has welded it on to me. I wonder, too, if the anger I feel so easily, so often, is now a part of who I am. Whoever that is.

The plot becomes even more inexplicable as I battle to keep my shifting mind focused on it and away from the clamorous chatter going on in my head. I end up understanding nothing of what is going on, and am terrified that someone will find me out.

The tube journey home is the worst of my life. They tip us all out at Baker Street, then again at Edgware Road. By the time the next District Line train shows up, I am frightened by how weak I feel. The train is full, of course, but I know I am in a seriously bad way. To my surprise, I hear myself say to a young man who is sprawling his long legs out into the gangway from the special seat reserved for the elderly or those with children, 'Can I sit there? I'm convalescent from brain surgery.' For a few seconds he carries on keeping time to the tinny music that I can just hear, coming out from his headphones. It's only from his manner when he makes way for me to sit down that I realise I must look as ill as I feel because, wired up as he is, he simply could not have heard what I said.

I can't continue pondering the psychological issues that the TV read-through threw up as, for the rest of the journey, I am taken over by the vicious pain in my head and the violent waves of nausea that accompany it. I no longer care if I'm sick on the tube floor. My ever-present worry of collapsing in public and having people walk round me is less fierce. I am past caring. I have the small comfort of having written my son's phone number on a piece of paper that's tucked inside my driving licence 'in case of emergency'. The only thing I want, apart from the sickness and the pain to stop, is not to have to do the walk home. By the time I have made my way feebly off the train and down the stairs to the pavement, I have nothing left at all. My head is empty. My body is no longer part of me. I am watching myself from somewhere far above. I want to lie down on the ground in the shade by the newsagent's stall. I have had enough. I give up.

CHAPTER SEVENTEEN

Help at Last

'You're a classic.'

'Sorry?'

'You're a classic—in your behaviour and emotional problems,' Mr Kitchen smiles.

I wipe another string of snot from my nose. The sobs are diminishing, but they still catch my breath and cause me to shudder as I breathe in. As I have just been recounting it— the injustice of Doc X's behaviour towards me in Warwickshire—it seems vividly present. There is no sound in the room apart from my quiet staccato breaths. Hard to believe that we're in the centre of London: the National

Hospital for Neurology and Neurosurgery.

'Depression is quite a common symptom after brain surgery. Lots of people get it.'

I am not mad. I feel vague, but strangely lightheaded, as if a weight has shifted imperceptibly somewhere. Depression is common.

My chest still aches with the rawness that has accompanied me for weeks, but in spite of it I want to get down on the floor and kiss this man's feet. Depression is common. The only thing that's stopping me doing the foot job is that I don't know how to move. I have not got a nerve in my body. I want to sit here in the cool, grey-slatted light of this sparse room and never move. I don't want to disturb this blissful rare calm.

'They did a very good job on you,' he says, holding up, then clamping to the board behind him, the by-now-familiar MRI scans of my brain. 'Mmm, very good,' he repeats. I smile weakly as if I share his interest and feel, ridiculously, that some of the approval could be for me. 'Look at this here,' he says, and points with great relish to what looks like a very fine curved kirby-grip that seems to be connecting two rather wiggly trunk roads on an Ordnance Survey map. It's always the bulge of the eyeballs, or the concave scoop that contains them, that I find disconcerting. That's what makes these rather uninteresting black and white and grey plates human. The bleed itself looks like ink squirted into a glass of water: its tentacles spread and curl in curiously pleasing swirls.

I do look. I am intrigued. Before, I was too scared to look. I feel a bit braver now, somehow. I have help. That's it. This man is going to help me. He's on my side. He isn't blaming me, or criticising.

'I have been very depressed,' I offer nervously, as if he's going to section me there and then.

'Depression's very common after brain surgery, as I said. It's the most invasive surgery of all.'

So it's OK that I'm not OK. I feel, at last, I have permission to feel dreadful and, of course, now I feel elated. Forget kneeling to kiss his feet. I want to lick the carpet before he steps on to it. 'I'm on anti-depressants,' I offer, as if admitting to a criminal tendency.

'Very sensible, until the serotonin levels in the brain readjust themselves.'

'Sensible' is far from the word I would use to describe the GP in the country, who still dominates my ever-growing hate list. But I have to admit to myself that the anti-depressants were her idea, as, apparently, was this hospital.

'I get these sort of twinges . . . well, it's not really dizziness. It's a tightness as if my brain is . . .' I look for a word. For a few seconds there are no words at all in my head. 'Fizzing.'

'Do you mean dizzy?'

Do I?

'No. It's a sort of zapping noise. I can actually hear it. Which is odd because I am deaf—well, I can't hear it—I mean, not with my ears, it's inside my head.' I'm talking too much again. The words are tumbling and jumbling out.

'We'll start to reduce the Neurontin slowly. Very slowly.'

How different is his quiet, assured way from that of Doc X and Mr Y. I feel safe with this man, although somewhere at the back of my mind I acknowledge that he seems very young to be a brain surgeon. Unless I'm older than I think. Time games again.

'Because I still could have a fit?' I ask, in my most reasonable voice. I want to say, 'Have you any idea what it's like not to know if you're going to fall down and twitch and dribble? It's terrifying.' I want to say, 'Have you any idea what having a fit in a rehearsal room would do to my working life?' But I don't. Somehow, some of the anger seems to have diffused.

'I never used to be a wimp,' I offer lamely. I was never a hypochondriac either. I never thought about my body at all. Somewhere, in a very secret place that I don't like to admit, I still think all this is my fault. My fault for driving my body too hard for years.

'I get so tired. I do nothing and I get so tired.' Just saying it makes me feel utterly depleted. I seem to have reached that bottom of places again. Now I'm hopeless. Tears sting the back of my throat yet again. I have the journey on the tube to face with two changes. It all seems suddenly impossible—facing the tube, the pushing and shoving, the noise, all the faces, the walk home from the station counting every step as I get nearer to the empty house. Dreaded self-pity. Where will that get me? I try all the usual sticks to bully myself out of it, my stepfather's rallying 'The more you cry, the less you'll pee,' but I can't rally even a shred of emotional muscle. I heave and shake with sobs that will make their way out.

'I'm so sorry,' I splutter. 'Sorry.' I've never said sorry so much in my life as I have this year. Why is that? 'I keep saying sorry.'

'Nothing to be sorry about. You're reacting like all brain patients. Tears and fatigue—'

'And cerebral irritation,' I add, knowing by now that calling it by its medical name, newly gleaned from the American information sheets, somehow lets my appalling tetchiness off the hook—at least in my own eyes. No one else's, that's for sure. With that thought comes its accompanying bubble of anger. It's better when I feel mad not sad about the friends who are no longer friends. At least it thwarts the tears and gives me a second to think. 'I just can't handle stress of any kind.'

'Well, no, and you won't be able to for a

254

good while yet.'

'How long?' I know, of course, that this question is as ridiculous as asking a gynaecologist how long labour will last.

'No two brain patients' recovery is the same. But you're a classic, as I said.'

'What?'

'A classic in your behaviour and emotional problems.'

I find I want to smile. This man isn't surprised by my behaviour. The only person in the world who isn't, including me. The stillness of the humid grey August afternoon seeps into the room once more. I want to smile, but it comes out as a sigh.

'Would you like some neuro-psychology rehab?' he asks, as I mop up the vanguard of another line of tears that have assembled from somewhere. It's the kindness. The kindness did it.

Neuro-psychology? I have no idea what it is. 'Yes, please,' I say, thinking it'll be good just to have someone to talk to. Someone to go to, to help me with this problem. This problem that I seem to have become. This problem whoever-she-is.

I must look a sight but I don't care. I wipe my eyes and clean up the residual snot, because I don't want this quiet, contained man to think, like Mr Y, that all actors are helpless, emotional creatures. I am all right now, aren't I? I ask myself. Even as I begin to think I am, a dread grows that the surges of emotion and helplessness are again reassembling their forces in the wings.

'I'm sorry I seem to be so weepy these days,' I offer, because that's what I think a normal person would say, but I tack on, in spite of myself, a nervous, pathetic laugh that makes me cringe inwardly.

'Oh, all quite normal,' says Mr Kitchen, sweeping it aside in that bright and breezy manner doctors survive on. A manner for which I now have a glimpse of understanding.

'What do I do about the MRI?'

'Oh you can have that when the two years are up.' Another sixteen months. The horizon widens.

'What about the insurance?'

'Oh, I'll write a letter to them to tell them you're still frail. You're a long way off going back to work.'

'I have ... four days ...'

'What?'

'Four days. Work ... Two days. With two days off in between. I'll only be actually working for an hour or so each day. There's a lot of sitting around on a film.'

'Film' sounds a very grand title for one episode of a TV series.

'Oh, that's good, settle into it gently.' No way of settling gently into eight performances a week in the theatre, I think ruefully. That part of my world is still out of reach.

'The insurance?' he continues.

'Insurance. Oh, yes . . . For the film.'

'Sometimes film companies want you to have a medical.'

Ruefully I recall the form that has to be filled in. It asks if you've been in hospital over the last five years. I wonder what 'Yes. Three and a half weeks in Intensive Care' would look like.

'Well, you're less of a risk than people walking around who don't know *what*'s going on inside *their* heads.' I feel comforted by his sureness. Then he says something like, 'Only twenty per cent of the half a per cent of people who *have* second aneurysms, have them . . .' I know he's dodging saying 'burst' ' . . . er, give trouble.'

Twenty per cent of half a per cent? The figures mean nothing to me. Figures never have done. But even I, mathematically challenged as I am, understand that this is very small.

'But the second aneurysm.'

'It's less than six millimetres, isn't it?' He makes that sound very small indeed.

I nod. Was it? Is it? I command myself to recall: Vinikoff operates at eleven. Patty's friend Marchosky operates at six. I'm trying to choose a happy medium for the size of mine when he says, 'Oh, I don't operate until it's one centimetre. Now, you go off and enjoy your holiday. Spain, you said?'

Did I? 'What shall I do about Doc X?'

'Ditch her. Enjoy Spain.'

'What?'

'You said you were going off to Spain for your holiday.'

'Oh, Ibiza, yes.'

'Do you want the rehab?'

'Yes.'

'Are you all right now?'

'Yes.'

I've just said yes more than I have for a very long time.

Spain. Off Neurontin. Well, off and on Neurontin.

I wonder what the Spanish is for 'epileptic fit'.

Ibiza. Yes. I wish I was out of the hot London traffic and there already. But, even more, I wish I'd cracked a joke about doing drugs and going clubbing.

CHAPTER EIGHTEEN

Brain and Scales

Back in the country I get the bike out, ostensibly to go food shopping, but I'm really on the lookout for some new clothes to take on holiday. It's not a proper holiday without something new to wear, and my backside isn't just behind, it's now at the sides and in front too since I've been sitting around so much. There are a couple of ladies' clothes shops in the nearest town. One is also a haberdasher's that is still stuck in the 1940s. It sells, among other oddities, those strips you sew under the shoulders of blouses and dresses so the bra straps don't show. They don't know the fashion world has come full circle. The other shop sells knife-sharp pleated skirts in fierce patterns that have matching blazers with alarming brass buttons at prices that are more than my week's food bill. So I'm not spoiled for choice. It's while I'm looking in these areas where I don't normally shop that I see it. In a sort of general-store window, among the pretend cut-glass vases and the pottery jam containers, complete with lids and spoons, sits the lion. I lurch off the bike, propel it to the nearest wall and dash into the shop. How much is that lion in the window . . .

'There's a lion in the window—how much is it, please?'

'Twelve poun',' says the old man behind the counter, who has a fine display of mutton-chop whiskers, small square-rimmed glasses and an imperturbable air. He comes out from behind the counter, his belt and braces adding to the Dickensian air, and slowly picks his way through the stuffed racks of toys, displays of seeds and the odd beachball. Twelve pounds is more than I wanted to pay.

Once the lion is in my hands I know it is mine. He is not as tatty as the one in the dream, but he has a fine mane that could be made to stick together in clumps. 'No need to wrap him up,' I say, 'I'll take him like this.' Then, feeling I have to tell the truth, I add, triumphant, 'He's not for a grandchild, he's for me.' The bell on the shop door tinkles, and someone in wellington boots and dungarees looks taken aback as a middle-aged woman edges past him clutching a lion, beaming.

At home the two are introduced to each other. I decide they will both guard my sleep. I also decide that I have had enough of the raw mother-son scenario. These two are father and daughter. With the still sensitive fingers of my left hand burrowed deep in the lion's fur, I make tracks slowly forwards and backwards until sleep catches me out. It's taken me fifty-five years and brain damage to replace, albeit in toy form, the father I know nothing about.

So, thanks to Mr Kitchen, I meet with Dr Miotto, neuro-psychologist, a slim, pretty blonde girl who dresses in stylish black trouser suits and, in spite of her Italian name, is Brazilian. Her grasp of English is astonishing. She uses several words I've never heard of. In fact, I've never heard of cognitive therapy and feel pretty scathing about it. I feel pretty scathing about most things most days, of course. If distress and anxiety are provoked by a fear or a trauma that goes way back into childhood, deal with the fear and trauma, don't just deal with the damn symptoms. In the weeks ahead I'm going to become more and more familiar with damn symptoms. Symptoms that I didn't know I have and don't know how to handle. Symptoms that don't always present themselves within the safe and understanding confines of the hospital either.

Getting to the neuro-psychology department is a brain test in itself, and that's after the cattle-truck jostling on the tube. Walking from Russell Square against a spiteful little September wind with teeth, I am slowed to a pace that is redolent of my speed at the end of the day, and it's only a quarter to ten. As I turn the corner to the main doors of the building I notice a sign on some railings leading down to a basement that says, 'Dizziness Clinic. This Way'. For a brief few seconds the whole day lightens. I am in a place where feeling spaced-out and head-zapped is the norm. I feel a spurt of energy and something that resembles joy. I walk up the steps eagerly.

There's a dauntingly huge reception area, with a large, ugly portrait of Princess Diana. I find it mesmerising and rather unsettling. Why is it there? Was she a patron of this hospital? Possibly. Would she have been a brain patient if she had survived that crash? Almost certainly. The real masterpiece, though, is a firmly worded notice on the reception desk that reminds patients that 'the staff will not tolerate aggressive or rude behaviour'. So they know about me. It's strangely comforting. Just let them try to be rude or aggressive to *me*, I retaliate inwardly. Eventually, after what seems an age of leaning on the reception desk, with the familiar bubbling inside of impatience, finally, in response to a telephone call, someone appears from the pavement outside and takes me out, then back into the building through a side entrance, a jumble of stairs, lifts, corridors, none of which I remember or take in. I follow meekly behind whoever this is—they have to stop several times to let me catch up. In the lift we go up to the second floor. I hold my head. My stomach lurches upwards, but my brain stays resolutely on the ground.

To my astonishment, I am offered a cup of coffee (decaf)—oh, of course, this is private medicine where they treat you like a person, not one of the herd. My sickness insurance is paying for this, at Mr Kitchen's instigation. I sip the coffee gratefully—it could be any tasteless hot drink, nothing new or lavish there then—while I skim through several glossy magazines with a difference. These are highly coloured, diagram-filled medical monthlies for the brain-crazed. There are alarming pictures of synaptic gaps with neurons in lurid red and green, cerebellums, in intestine-like folds of creamy yellow, medullas and cortexes in purples and blues. The brain looks as colourful and chaotic as Times Square. And that's only from the outside. The colours jump off the page at me. I feel I must study these pictures and learn all about the brain that I can. *Now. Quick.*

But the tube journey so early in the morning in the rush-hour crowds has left me nothing to concentrate with. I look around. It's a bit like a slightly seedy hotel. There are many closed doors along the corridor I'm sitting in. I wonder if behind every one of them is someone as angry, as defiant, as beaten and bewildered as whoever this person is that I call me. I realise that I am anxious because I don't know what I'm going to find out.

So on Friday 8 September, almost eight months to the day, I find a helpful, quietly spoken, kindly accomplice. She listens to my jumbled accounts of distress, my ramblings about my estranged son. 'You can't deal with anyone who is emotionally needy, and he obviously can't deal with you.'

My world lurches. I am very near to being overwhelmed. She pushes a box of Kleenex towards me. 'Expect nothing from him,' she says quietly.

I want to say, 'But he's all I've got.' It sounds so pathetic, even as a silent thought in my head.

She lifts the box nearer to me and urges me

to take one. I wonder if they get their tissues wholesale. I wonder how many they get through in a week. I take several and swallow hard again and again. Just as well I can't speak. 'Most people are monitored immediately.'

Why didn't the French tell me this? I wonder. Why was I just tipped out of the hospital with a packet of paracetamol and Neurontin as if everything in the frontal lobe was lovely? Mustn't be ungrateful, they saved my life. A life that is becoming less prickly and uncomfortable the longer I spend in this rather bare room with this lovely girl.

'Loss of friends. Is that er . . . normal?' I manage.

'Yes, it's quite common.'

So I'm not mad.

I want to line them all up and shout at them, 'You sods made me iller.' This swing from despair to defiance is giddy. That is mad.

'Are there many patients who convalesce alone?'

'Not many. Families, of course, are the first to detect the changes. Tiredness is the major factor after surgery, that and irritability. And difficulty in handling stress.'

I seem to have major, major factors. 'My job is all stress.'

'Most executives reduce their hours when they go back to work.'

I've never thought of my work as stuff executives are made on, but I suppose it is—in the real world—in terms of leading a company, having responsibility for the growth, the speed of a play, keeping a weather eye on how it changes and develops. But how can I reduce my hours? I'm not *that* sort of executive. I can't call the tune like that. A performance is a performance. Can't just do a bit of Act Two. So the theatre's still out of reach, then.

'It's the third biggest killer.'

'Cancer?'

'Yes.'

'Heart-attacks?'

'Yes.'

'Strokes?'

'And aneurysms.'

I trot out my motto to Dr Miotto: 'Stroke patients can be *seen* to have had damage. We can't. It's like being deaf. Blind people get all the sympathy because—'

Very gently she continues. I feel like a child who doesn't know when to stop talking. I have a clear glimpse of my chatting on and on to fill the uncomfortable silences between my mother and my foster-mother on the rare occasions they met.

'Subarachnoid haemorrhage, which is what you had . . . The brain is in a kind of sac.' Effectively, and upside down for my benefit, she draws a head. 'The brain and the spinal stem are protected by three layers of membrane. One of these is called arachnoid.' For the first time I take a real interest in the

265

enemy. 'You had a middle cerebral-artery haemorrhage, didn't you?' I nod: it sounds like a vaguely familiar pattern of words. She refers momentarily to some papers she has beside her on the desk. They must have come from Mr Kitchen. I feel hugely cherished. Then she draws a little balloon bulging from a stem. A bit like a ripe fruit growing straight from it, no stalk. 'And they clip it like this.' She neatly separates the bulge from the stem. Inwardly I flinch, yet at the same time I am jolted into offering new thanks to the guardian angels and, wondering which is east, shove some more in the direction of Paris and the valiant Dr Vinikoff.

'It's not the same as a stroke, is it?'

'No, a stroke is caused by a blockage of blood, which may cause a weakness down one side where the brain was deprived of blood. Here, the brain is flooded with blood.'

'They're the people who get the sympathy—the understanding, I mean—because they can be *seen* to have suffered, to have . . . a problem.' I am ashamed to acknowledge how near I am to tears. It's a very acute welling up of a sense of injustice done to me by the so-called friends. Then, chastened, I remember that I didn't know any of this earlier, so what right have I to blame them? My foster-mother was quick to judge others and I learned well at her knee. Angry with myself, I wipe away the offending drops roughly.

Discreetly she tidies the pile of papers on her desk. 'I think we've done enough for one day.' I look at my watch. An hour has gone by. I cannot believe a whole hour has gone by. 'It's eleven o'clock,' I say, unconvinced.

'Do you have trouble with short-term memory?'

'What?' She is about to reply when I say, 'Who are you again?' She giggles.

'Do you lose track of what you're doing?'

'Well . . .' I search consciously for a memory and, as if playing hide and seek, my mind empties instantly. I sigh, exasperated.

'Don't worry—it doesn't matter.'

'Yes, it *does*,' I say sharply. 'I *have* to remember. I'm an actor. No memory, no job.' I have raised my voice and it is tinged with desperation.

'We should stop now anyway, and you're getting tired.'

I want to say, 'No, I'm not!' like a truculent child, but I am. Truculent and tired. Tired to my bones. Again. I am overcome with helplessness and the accompanying waterworks. I blurt out, 'I can find myself in the garden emptying the b-b-bathroom ru-u-ubbh-bish bin, no idea how I got there or why, then when I g-g-g-go upstairs I find that I was cleaning the bathroom mirror, because there's a can of polish and a cloth, and the Hoover is in another room.' The tears make it sound a vital pastime. I realise this gives an untypical

267

picture both of me and my rural slum. Or, rather, my attitude to housework, which is largely leave it till someone visits and it becomes an embarrassment that has to be dealt with. How small and domestic my life is now, considering that I won the Nobel Prize for Chemistry (and Physics) as Marie Curie, ruled most of twelfth-century France as doughty Alienor of Aquitaine, charmed crusty, confirmed bachelor C.S. Lewis and stood up to the high table at Magdalen as feisty Joy Davidman, led the French to war as Saint Joan and got through more men, drugs and drink than you could shake a stick at as Piaf.

'Do you have trouble with your words?'

I am crammed full of them.

I remember the Shakespeare in St Louis and Montréal. And, guiltily, the lines I'll have to learn for the TV film that somehow I haven't told her about. It'll be all right. I am, after all, going on holiday first.

'No,' I say defensively and boast, 'I've learned Gerard Manley Hopkins.' This is lost on a Brazilian. 'English poet. Very hard. Lots of big words.' I have lapsed into almost pidgin English, which makes me snort with laughter. I wipe away the tears, wishing I was bemused by this ludicrous behaviour.

'I want you to keep a chart of what you do each day. On a piece of paper you put things like, "Ten a.m., read the newspaper. Twelve, walk round the park. One p.m., have lunch,"

268

that kind of thing.' I feel instantly guilty that I have not walked through the park since . . . I can't remember when.

'I can't remember,' I say out loud.

'And please make a chart or a list of how frustrating certain experiences are.'

'Frustrating?' I roll the word around my mind as if I'd never heard it before.

'Yes, you know, how irritable you get if you're, say, kept waiting in a queue in a shop, six out of ten, for example, for a bus, two out of ten.'

'Oh, yes.' So that's what it is. I just thought it was me being my usual impatient self. Only more so. Impulsive. Yes. Bees in bonnet. Piano. Andes. Overwhelmed. Volatile. Oversensitive. Yes yes yes. Only more so.

'Would you like to do a neuro-psychology test?' I try to pull myself together: just getting home on the tube will be a fight to the bitter end. How can I possibly manage a test now? She senses the change in my attitude and says, smiling, 'No, no, not now. You must go home and rest. Do nothing for the rest of the day.' What a ridiculous idea, I think. I've got the leaves to sweep up, all the mail to collect to take back to the cottage to answer, about six phone calls to make. I have to do these things when I'm in London. That's what London's *for*. It justifies my coming here. Somehow I don't dare say any of this. Like an alcoholic, I feel I'm hiding the whisky behind the fridge. I have to work, I just have to. If I don't, the few threads of a career that I do have may all unravel even more. Besides, I love my job.

'It's very tiring travelling.'

'What?' I've lost the thread.

'When the brain is in motion it takes a lot of energy to stay balanced and deal with all the stimuli. We'll book another appointment for later in the day next time, so you don't have to travel through the rush-hour.'

In a blinding flash I realise I have never thought of that. Such a simple thing. How stupid of me. 'I'm stupid. Never thought—'

'Well, you didn't have to before, did you? That's quite normal, but now you do. You have to think of how to make things easy for the person that you are *now*.'

So it *is* different. *I am* different. *Who* am I? I am sick of sounding, even to myself, like a teenager with an identity crisis. I have the spots to go with it too.

'So would you like to do a neuro-psychology test when you come back from your holiday, then?'

'Yes. Yes,' I say eagerly, thinking of how it will have to wait till after the filming too.

'Then we will have an idea of what your cognitive deficits are.' I have no idea what 'cognitive deficits' means. She smiles and says, 'And would you like to read some material about SAHs?'

'Yes, yes, please.' What a good student.

What a good patient. I make myself sick.

She turns to her filing cabinet and hands me ten or so pages stapled together under the blistering title 'Quality of life and cognitive deficits after subarachnoid haemorrhage' from the *British Journal of Neurosurgery, 1995.* Great beach reading.

> The incidence of aneurysmal subarachnoid haemorrhage [what I had] is about one in 10,000 per year in the general population. Out of these 60% can be regarded as functional survivors (i.e. can talk and walk). Faced with this large number of people who suffer SAH mostly in the middle of their lives, the question of the *quality* of their life becomes increasingly important. In neurological outcome research, scales refer only to the *physical* functional level and *dependency* of the patient. They do not assess sufficiently all the *relevant* aspects of *quality* of life. Many patients report such diffuse complaints as irritability, personality change, loss of interests and emotional disturbances.

Here I'm happy to be one of the many. I'm certainly relieved. Relieved to be irritable, changed and disturbed.

In a retrospective study of 58 patients after SAH examined 1-5 years after the event for their quality of life, including a neuro-psychological examination, cognitive deficits were found in:

visual short-term memory, 46%
reaction-time task ranging from 31% to 65%
verbal long-term memory, 28%
concentration, 5-13%
language, 11%

The quality of life was reduced in the SAH patients according to a self-rating scale:

in motivation, 50%
interests, 47%
mental capacity, 47%
free-time activities, 52%
social relationships, 39%
concentration, 70%
fine motor co-ordination, 25%
sleep, 47%

A further 77% of the patients reported *more frequent headaches* since their SAH. *Depression* was found in 30%. *Life satisfaction was significantly reduced* in 37% whereas 48% suffered from *increased emotional swings*, and in 41% motivation was significantly reduced. *Negative job consequences*, like loss of job or demotion, were reported by 16% of the patients investigated, and an additional 15% had been retired.

I don't like the word 'retired' one tiny bit.

Assessment of personality disturbances, depression and working capacity. For assessing the emotional state of the SAH patients, the FPI-R (a German Standard Personality form) was used.
   This personality inventory consists of the following 12 bipolar subscales:
(1) life satisfaction vs life dissatisfaction;
(2) social responsibility vs *selfishness;*
(3) ambition vs loss of motivation;
(4) social insecurity vs assertiveness;
(5) sensitivity vs calm;
(6) *aggressiveness* vs inaggressiveness;
(7) strained vs stable;
(8) bodily complaints vs health;
(9) bodily concern vs no bodily concern;
(10) openness vs social desirability;
(11) extraversion vs introversion;
(12) *emotional lability* vs emotional stability.

I read and reread all this several times. I certainly have a lot of (2), (6), and (12). Then I think, Well, I always had, but now it's more so. I notice there's no sense of humour on the list. The scale is German.

In order to assess quality of life an ad hoc scale for patients self-rating containing 11 items and a parallel version for rating the complaints of the patients by their life companions were used.

I am a non-starter on the life-companions bit.

The items included have a face-validity and were selected for complaints in those areas which are typical for patients with brain damage:
(1) life insecurity in social relationships;
(2) reduction in free-time activities;
(3) reduction in mental capacity;
(4) reduction in concentration;
(5) reduction of interest for daily problems (indifference);
(6) loss of motivation;
(7) sensory-motor fine co-ordination;
(8) sleeping problems;
(9) patients' subjective feelings of lacking information about their illness;
(10) headaches;
(11) a feeling of bodily imperfection.
(The response to items (9), (10), (11) were counted separately. The items were set up according to a five-point Likert scale. Only such subjective complaints were regarded as substantial if the patient reported at least a fair degree of impairment.)

Well, I thought, I don't think the tube can be counted as 'social relationships'. So I have a lot of (3), (4), and (8), a fair amount of (10), none at all of (5), and the rest are don't-knows. And don't care. Oh, no, that's number (5). I'd never thought about brain damage before. I'd joked about it. Every time someone commented on their bad memory I came in on cue with 'Well, I've had brain surgery. What's your excuse?' My brain, I had assumed, had been repaired. 'Impaired' was something altogether new and scary.

> Patients with cerebral damage may not be able to perceive their deficits reliably. Therefore it is useful to rate the problems of their life-companions. To ensure that the partners were able to judge the patients reliably, only those questionnaires were included when both had lived together under one roof for at least 5 years.

So this selfish, aggressive, functional survivor with a non-shared roof took herself off on holiday, to walk, read, sit in the sun and, please God, sleep.

CHAPTER NINETEEN

Brain in Spain, TV and Start Again

It looked as if it was going to be a short-lived break as, on arrival, no taxi would take me from the airport to the Old Town where my friend's little flat is. A new traffic scheme had been introduced to limit the amount of cars climbing the winding, narrow, cobbled lanes up to the ruins of the medieval castle at the top and even taxis had to have a pass. I stood in the queue in the sticky heat in the late-afternoon light with my ridiculously huge suitcase packed with things I wouldn't use and, yes, I cried. A couple behind me took pity on me and offered to share their taxi, which arrived complete with the necessary pass. They had come, as they came twice a year, to escape the cold and damp in England as he, the husband, had MS. We talk openly and freely as people do who are ill. It is a strong bond. I envied him his wife but not his wheelchair.

My constant companions, apart from the eight books for ten days, are, it would seem, colours. Unaware, I have draped over the backs of the four chairs round the little table in the sitting room-cum-kitchen in Cherry and Mike's flat a pink dress, a lavender dress, a dark blue-green beach wrap and a turquoise T-shirt. I can feel the energy that comes off these colours. It is almost tangible. I feel cheered and comforted by them when I arrive back after the long slog up the cobbled hill and narrow dank alleys from the port. The deep purple of the bougainvillaea that spills over a startlingly white wall on my daily path to Maria's small, dark store, which smells of olive oil and candles, makes me catch my breath and stare. I write in my journal, 'Everything is so acute.' My brain, which I can still feel, makes its zapping noises more frequently now, even when I am not turning my head. I suspect it is getting used to the lower dose of anti-epilepsy drug, and my eyes are getting used to the bright lights dancing on the water. Apart from the sun, it doesn't really feel like a holiday. It's just another series of days to get through, hoping that no major pain strikes. I manage a siesta most afternoons. It gives my head a break from its hat and the beating sun. Often I am alarmed by the deafening buzz and whine of the Vespas that the local youngsters ride, swooping up and down the hill. After they have passed and I have cowered from the noise, I indulge in the few rude words I know in Spanish and, like the cranky old lady I have become, I shake my fist at them.

I say a long goodbye to the sun on my last day. Longer than I planned. The flight is delayed by two, then three, then four hours. It means that even with an expensive taxi ride I won't be home in London until two or three in the morning. The level of exhaustion I know I will then feel frightens me. Like every other person in the airport I use my mobile phone. But, unlike all the other adults speaking, I sound like a six-year-old. I beg my son to be at home to meet me. He agrees. He knows I know he can hear the fear.

I have some trouble adjusting to standing in a Berkshire lane at eight o'clock in the morning in a grey frizzy wig, aware of a heavy dew on the chrysanthemums and Michaelmas daisies in cottage gardens. Some leaves have already begun to turn golden on the silver birch trees nearby, and our breath is just perceptible on the morning air as we drink our location coffee in its ghastly polystyrene cups. I feel elated to be working. Overjoyed, too, that I can remember my lines. Grateful for the seat that is proffered at the end of every short take.

I am triumphant that my professional self still knows what to do. I hit my marks—more instinct than conscious accuracy because if I look down I feel dizzy; I give lines off-camera for others' close-ups. I never lose the place where we are, but I have been hurtled down the M40 at six o'clock in the morning by student drivers for whom speed is of the essence. By the second day I am wiped out before I start. Of course, having to put my hands flat on the floor as the ballet dancer my character was, doesn't help, especially as I get cheap laughs by chatting to the cameraman in that position. Even after the two-day break, in which I am good for nothing, the suspicion of a major head pain grows into a full blown relentless hammering just behind the scar, so that by the last day, no longer caring about who knows it or who sees me, I spend most of the day and night of shooting curled up on a pile of coats on one of the beds in the cottage we're using for my character's house. I work, tanked up on painkillers, for about ten minutes that day, but I am kept till midnight to complete a thirty-second night shot. On the way home in the car, whose driver I have implored to go slowly, I stretch out on the back seat holding my head, groaning at every bump in the road, sick with pain.

Those four days of work set me back . . . six months? Not that the diary shows it. Hair appointments, teaching the odd class, getting the video-machine collected and fixed. Visiting my theatre club in Bristol. Recording a voiceover for BBC TV (need the money). Taking my son out to dinner (spending the money)—I should have stayed in bed. But bed isn't part of the life I know. Besides, bed is a hard place to be when you live alone and are in pain. Anyway, only really ill people need to stay in bed. After all, it's only a headache. Or is it?

At least I compromise on the busyness, with a work interview that crops up suddenly. An interview for another TV job. I am thrilled. Work's still coming in. This is like it used to be before . . . before . . . What do I say? Do I talk about being ill? The director himself helps me achieve the compromise by kindly offering to call round to my house on his way in to work to save me having to get to his office in Soho during the morning rush-hour. I've had a bit of practice at performing, so at nine o'clock one October morning I do an impersonation of a woman feeling fine, serving coffee and biscuits to this director while he sets up a video-camera in her sitting room. It feels very odd. It is. Odd. I have never been interviewed on video for a TV job in my own sitting room, in which, as it happens, I haven't sat properly for months. I feel almost a stranger in my own home. So I enlarge my performance into a woman who takes this in her stride, as if it were the most natural thing in the world to be filmed having my breakfast and talking to myself.

I get the job. Odd. I can't believe it. Even odder that I mentioned in passing that I had been rather ill, but they still want to go with me. An icy finger uncurls in my guts when I think, Insurance. I'll have to have a medical for the film insurance. Mr Kitchen will help.

Mr Kitchen the neuro-surgeon said he would help. It'll be all right. It's all happened a bit too quickly for me, but that's the nature of the work beast for the self-employed. I've promised to do a charity performance in the village church to raise money for a local voluntary service the day before the filming starts, but that won't matter. It's on a Sunday evening, after all. It'll just be a question of not filming first thing Monday morning to allow me time to travel to London and settle into living here at home again. Better learn a lesson from the last time. Better ask for a proper driver who won't hurtle me at ninety miles an hour and swing my head round corners. Best to ask. My agent and I agree that care is the name of the game. Slowly, at first, I begin to get used to the idea of being back in the swing of things. Being in a TV series. A series, what's more, that is well written—and funny too. A rare beast indeed. I become exultant. I think, in my most jubilant moments, well, it was nothing, this illness. Look how quickly I am over it. It turns out that, fortuitously, the job has a generous salary attached. I am euphoric. I fantasise about spending all the money on white or cream furniture for the new flat. I will have everything new. New life, new flat, new car (when I feel like driving in London).

I am so excited that even the prospect of giving up the little pension—I'll be back at work full time—isn't a problem. Back at work.

Back to 'normal'. I allow me to say that word to myself, but I don't know what it means. I know I don't know what normal is—was. Back to before my son was born? Back to before I was on the treadmill of being a single parent? That's half a lifetime away. Exactly half. Exactly twenty-eight years. I can't expect to feel the same at fifty-six as I did at twenty-eight. Can I? What *can* I expect to feel? As I stand, some days later, in a costumier's, being fitted for ten or twelve outfits I will need for the six-week shoot, having to make quite subtle judgements about the character with each item of clothing, each scarf, blouse, pair of shoes, I slowly realise the unpalatable answer to my question.

The designer and I work well together: we are sympathetic to the character and to each other's understanding of it. This is film, the scrutiny of the camera in close-up can be fierce, so the clothes choices mustn't caricature the character. I must wear *them*, they mustn't be allowed to wear *me*. The woman who runs this vast emporium of garments and accessories knows, surprisingly, that I have been ill. She is ever solicitous with coffee, which of course I shouldn't really be drinking, and encouraging me to sit down between trying on different outfits, while she and her assistant disappear time and time again into the bowels of the building and search one more time among the hundreds of rails of clothes for just the right cardigan or skirt to complete an outfit. There is a damp, musty smell that pervades all places where clothes that have been worn are stored, and this place is no exception. The coffee sits uncomfortably in my excited, nervous stomach. I try to force down a banana, which I've had the presence of mind to bring with me, but it is heavy-going. As the afternoon progresses, the slightly cheesy smell in the air becomes unpleasantly insistent.

Recounting the illness—they want to know all the horrors, and I am a willing storyteller— while at the same time concentrating on the myriad short scenes this character has, scenes that are second nature to the designer as she's been working on this project for months, becomes increasingly hard. I feel slightly dizzy. I become confused. I get the order of certain scenes wrong. I have, after all, only read through the six episodes briefly. I don't really know my way round this. I mustn't let them see that.

What I seriously need to know is what the shooting schedule is like so that I know how much time I have off. Time in which I can put my feet up in my van and rest. But no one seems to have a schedule. So near the start of filming and no one seems to know what the first day's work is. That worries me. Rest. When can I rest? I become more and more reluctant to leave the safety of the bentwood

283

chair to stand up and try on a new outfit. Reluctant? Damn bad-tempered. The frustration level is off the scale. I become increasingly irritated by the rows of pins in a skirt or blouse that catch me and scratch me as I take garments off and put others on. I feel hot and bothered like a querulous child. I want to go home. Now. It's odd how at one moment I'm all right and then suddenly, as if all the sand has run out of an egg-timer, I'm far from all right. Empty. I can't wait to get home and lie down. But the time for rest has long passed. I know, too, it will be a long time before I stop hurting, before my body stops telling me I am ill. But I choose not to listen.

After an interminable minicab ride home, I share my anxiety about the performance in the church and the lack of shooting schedule with my agent, who promises to look into it and who always does what she says. Way past being aware of my behaviour, and the havoc several glasses of wine have wreaked, I ring the production office myself. The initial response, in a glowing Sharon/Tracy voice, is 'How do you spell your name?'

My confidence is in shreds. My temper past red alert. When I manage to extract the shooting information from the imbecile who, quite patently, has never worked on a film before, I realise, to my horror, from her mangled description that I am in the first shot at 8 a.m. on Monday morning. The convolutions of getting from the church after a performance that won't finish at least until 10 p.m., or going with who'll be driving to London that night, or getting a minicab from the cottage to London the next day at dawn before the other gazillion drivers hit the M40 or, better still, getting the film company to pick me up, but how to explain where the cottage is, all prove too much for my whacked-out brain. I try, somewhere between shouting and crying but mostly shouting, to make it clear that I simply can't let the Voluntary Service charity down, the posters have been printed, tickets have been sold, I have promised. Sharon/Tracy interjects, with her sing-song, 'Shall I say you won't be comin' in that Monday mornin', then?'

I gasp. You turn up to film if you're dying. Each minute on a film set costs thousands and thousands of pounds. No one is ever late. I can feel the chaos in that production office. It clings to me. It grates me raw. I feel like I did as a kid playing street games, Please, Mr Farmer, may I cross your golden river?' when in my dash to the other side of the road I fell and hit my middle on the kerb. Then, as now, I am winded.

I can't handle it at all. I blurt down the phone to the agent, gasping to get breath into my body as I whine and howl. She is brilliant. Calm and sensible, she reassures me that she will insist on a level of care and consideration for me, below which they Must Not Fall.

For a while the heaving, blubbering lump of incompetence that I have become walks round the kitchen eating whatever I find in my hand from the fridge. Then I have the brilliant idea of ringing the director and explaining the problem.

I start with 'I can't cope. I can't cope with the production office.'

He starts and finishes me with, 'Well, we'd better give the job to someone else.'

I scream out loud. I go on screaming. I beat my head with my hands.

The next day I have lost the best TV job I've had in years and twenty thousand pounds.

Patricia, in whose home I beg sanctuary that night, says, 'You really shouldn't mention that you've been ill. It was nine months ago. People don't remember. Get on with your life. That girl's job was on the line. She had to get you there on Monday morning. Don't keep talking about being ill.' I hug the big toy lion that I have brought with me, and recoil from all this harsh truth. But it is the truth. How lucky I am to have a friend who doesn't bullshit me. I make a mental note not to mention brains or haemorrhages again. Never. Ever. Or being ill. Never. Ever. Waiting for over an hour for my staccato breathing to subside and for the two sleeping pills to deaden my galloping brain, I hear a small voice inside me say, 'But I *am* ill.'

286

CHAPTER TWENTY

Brain Test

The neuro-psychology test starts at two o'clock. In spite of recalling what the American analyst said not to do, I *do* pull myself up by my bootstraps. I muster my forces as if I were beginning a first night. This, after all, is a competition. I have to do well. I have to do the best I can. New-me versus old-me.

There is a book of photographs with a different face on every page. Dr Miotto flicks through it quickly and I have to say when I recognise a face I've seen before. She reads out a long list of quite complicated words, and a variety of choices of meanings and I have to select the one I think correct. 'Postpone. Alternative. Haphazard. Intermittent . . .' I am intrigued by the significance and the juxtaposition of the words. No, no, that's not *the point.*

'If two apples cost thirty-five pence how much change will you have from a pound?'

Inwardly I groan. I could never do this kind of sum at primary school when I was nine, let alone at fifty-six after brain surgery. Then there are rows and rows of upright dashes—| | | | | | | | | | | | |; I have to see how quickly I can strike a line through each of them while she times me on a stop-watch. This is almost fun. I just wish I could make my hand, which is getting a bit sticky, move faster.

I have to put a circle round similar words arranged anyhow on a page. My eyes flick up and down and across and backwards. After two hours she asks if I would like a break.

'No, *no.* I have to k-k-keep going. I must keep g-g-going. I want to g-g-go on.'

Some time and several exercises later, she empties a box of wooden white and red coloured squares and triangles on to the table, then hands me a sheet of paper with many different formations of squares and triangles on it. 'Copy this pattern,' she says, pointing to one.

I can see the overall shape, but I can't work out if the pointed bit is made of two triangles back to back or a square with a triangle against it. I turn the triangle round. I pick up a square. I stare blankly at the page. Nothing is going on in my head at all.

'Try this one,' she says helpfully, pointing to another pattern. I start off eagerly, then am flummoxed by the number of squares in the pattern. Are they building blocks of squares? Or which ones have triangles added to them? I can't. None of it makes any sense at all. I put my head in my hands and weep and weep and weep. Dr Miotto gets up and hugs me. I cling to her for fear she will stop.

My hopes are high. Dr Miotto is in my life, I am not dealing with this thing—this monster—alone any more. I have another flat to view, which is slightly further down the road from the other two, but it has a garden. (So much for the dream flat's balcony and window-boxes.) It's also being managed by a woman estate agent, which is something else in its favour. Although it is a grey November day I have decided to make a day of it. Give myself a treat. I plan to walk from the tube in Sloane Square down to Battersea Bridge, taking some lunch with me as I tend to get faint, these days, if I don't eat. If I see some clothes or books that take my fancy, well, I might just treat myself. Shopping has become my major social pastime. It's not to meet people that I shop. I can barely tolerate the crowds and the brutish music. I look at the colours, bright shiny things, such a variety. I feed on them.

There is, of course, a queue at the tube ticket desk, it being a Monday morning, and the automatic ticket machine is again closed down. The queue is barely moving. It is only when I stand still that I become aware of just how much energy it takes to keep upright. I tire quickly. Everyone ahead of me is apparently buying a lifetime's worth of tickets, the movement in the queue is so imperceptible. The frustration pendulum begins to move and make itself felt.

I say to the girl in front of me, 'I have been

seriously ill, may I?' vaguely indicating the place ahead of her.

'Wha' yoo say?' She barely speaks English.

'Ill—me,' I shout, stabbing ridiculously at my own chest. The man in front of her moves sharply aside too, as if I have something contagious. At the head of the queue a question is asked, answered, and another contented customer walks away. There is a rustle of discomfort in the line that has rapidly assembled behind me. I feel I ought to say, 'It's only brain damage, it's not catching.' Is that mad? It's only the fact that two people ahead of me walk away together that distracts me from speaking. Suddenly I find myself at the ticket office. I am about to speak when a man with a long grey pigtail emerging from underneath his uniform cap says from behind the man selling tickets, 'Right, that's it. He's got to have a break. Get your tickets from the machine.' I am about to explode with impatience as I turn to explain that the machine in question isn't goddamn working when I hear a distant showering of coins. A few tinny rumbles and coughs from inside the machine and half the queue behind me rushes to assemble in front of it.

'Please could I have a ticket? I've not been well,' I say to the broad-faced man in the ticket office, who just happens to be black.

'Did you hear what I said?' Pigtail's voice has now risen a notch or two and is very abrasive. 'He hasn't had a break since five this morning.'

'I've had brain surgery.' I sound and feel pathetic.

'Where d'you want to go?' says the ticket man quietly.

'Sloane Square,' I say, hearing my voice resound in the concrete and tiled ticket hall, wishing I didn't sound so well spoken. Wishing I was going anywhere but Sloane Square.

'Return?'

'I don't care if you have had brain surgery, *he* hasn't had a break since five this morning.' He is now shouting. I push my ten-pound note across.

I am hot. There is a distinct unease among the rest of the stragglers in the queue. I collect the ticket and the change with some difficulty and turn to go.

'Is good 'e 'elp,' says the girl behind me.

'What?'

'Is good 'e 'elp,' she says, pointing at the ticket man.

'Good's got nothing to do with it,' I snap. 'It's called being a decent human being.' I don't know who the person is who comes out with these things. Though they are true.

I head for the stairs. Behind me I hear, 'I feel sorry for you, you know, I really do.' Pigtail is following me. 'No, no, I don't,' he says, as if correcting himself.

Quietly I say, 'I'm sure you don't, young

291

man.'

'Just because you've bloody had bloody brain surgery's no reason to be rude.' He is in full stride, coming up the stairs beside me.

I don't know why I can't unhook myself from this but I can't. 'I wasn't rude.'

He jumps the last step and turns on the platform to confront me. My knees feel like they are fizzing.

'I wasn't rude.'

Everything I say seems to enrage him. I want to say, 'I was brought up in the working class. I had to have free school dinners.' That's the truth of it, even though it seems mad. Is it mad? This wouldn't be happening to me if I wasn't mad.

'Just because you've had bloody brain surgery doesn't mean you can be rude to people,' he bellows at me. People further down the platform turn to see where the noise is coming from. A train bends its way round a curve in the track down the line. It takes an age to get to the platform. Time stands still. I am going to get on it wherever it is going. The doors open and I get on. So does he.

'You and your bloody brain surgery,' he says, swinging himself round towards me by a strap above his head, 'doesn't mean you can be rude to people.' I am full of dread that this heckling is going to pursue me for the entire journey. I can't stop my hands shaking.

'I wasn't rude,' I repeat, and in case anyone

292

listening thinks he might be right, I add, '*You* were rude to *me*.'

I tighten my grip on the rail beside me as I hear the doors begin to close. In a flash he is through them, out on the platform, still shouting and waving his arms in my direction as the train pulls out of the station. Sweat is running down my neck. I loosen my scarf. The carriage is almost empty. There are a couple of schoolboys, intent on some pocket game, a few workmen and a woman who turns to smile at me wryly. I want to scream, 'What the hell are you smiling about?' I can't, though, because a hot knife is burning as it turns in my back and I am winded from the kick in my chest.

What is it about this new me that seems to attract this treatment? Why are they drawn to me? Madness must have a special smell. I sniff at my armpits. Well, if I am mad I can do anything. A whole variety of entertaining options entice. I do smell. I smell of fear. And feel like Rip Van Winkle.

If this is the world now, I have no place in it.

There is a biting wind on Albert Bridge. I had the bridge wrong. It's not Battersea. It's Albert. How can I have got the bridge wrong? This is the only other street I have ever wanted to live on. I look up at the boulders of dark clouds scudding along in the grey sky. I feel as if the greyness has permeated into my head. Or, rather, my head has drifted up. I have no head. It is full of sky. There is a space where my head should be. Eat, I must eat. That might connect my head to my shoulders again. I lodge the coffee I've just bought on a ledge between me and the bridge and shove my lunch into my mouth. I am ravenous. I eat faster than I can swallow, helping it down with burning gulps of hot tastelessness. I stare down into the choppy brown churning water. Several runners pass. Some of them glance at me. I look up at the delicate ironwork tracery of this bridge that I love, as if this were the perfect day to be taking in such an idyllic view. It begins to rain. I pack up clumsily, showering rye breadcrumbs and splashes of coffee over my hands and mac, face into the wind and the long stretch of road ahead of me. From the edge of my vision, I can see that the nylon fur trim around my hood has become matted with rain.

By the time I reach the number in the road that corresponds to the estate agent's now soggy information sheet, I am at the very end of it. It would have been better to start from here. There's a joke there somewhere, I think, but I can't think of it. I can't think. There is a large murderous-looking motorbike parked rather haphazardly across the Victorian tiled path that leads up to the front door. Nailed to the wall at the side is the estate agent's sign.

Steps, which give on to a concrete area, lead down to the basement front door. Just above it are a few dusty, spiky plants. They would have been dusty but the rain has gouged circular frets in the dust. I wait in the drizzle, listening to water dripping from a pipe somewhere.

A small car draws up and a much made-up lady of a certain age gets out and heads towards me, keys jangling ahead of her. I greet her with, 'If I'd known it was a basement flat, I wouldn't have come. I've been ill. I don't want to live in a basement.'

'It's a garden flat,' she replies, with barely a start in her response, or a hiccup in her movement towards me.

'You can call it what you like,' I go on, 'but any flat that has bars at the window and the ground starting half-way up it is a basement. I wish your office had been honest with me.'

'This is the only window with bars on it,' she replies smoothly, and opens the front door.

Once inside the small hallway I look to my right, into what is obviously the main bedroom. I see that not only is it wall-to-bare-wall high-tech Japanese, but this is Not For Me. I wouldn't even want to die here, I think. Then I catch myself out. No jokes about that any more. The kitchen is in the corridor further on and looks like the cockpit of a plane. All the gadgets and equipment are on one side. It's a place you pass through. It is not somewhere you can cook while you talk to

295

friends sitting round a table drinking wine, which for me is the best way of cooking. Beyond this is a room that has one woodchip wall painted a startling but undeniable gold. My reaction must be evident because she turns to me and says, rather smugly, 'A designer for Armani lives here.'

It's now my turn to be nonplussed. 'Armani designs clothes not buildings.'

'No, but you know what I mean—'

'No, I don't. I don't give a damn about labels.'

She opens a door in this room that leads out on to the back steps. To the left is what I suppose used to be the coalhouse. Inside, snugly arranged, are the washing-machine and the dryer. The rain splats down on to me as it would if I had a bundle of dry clothes. I point up the stairs towards the garden, which stretches quite a distance and is abundant with flowering shrubs and several small but well-established trees. I ask what I presume is a rhetorical question: 'The garden isn't shared with anyone, is it?'

'Oh, this isn't your garden. Your garden is at the front.'

That does it. I laugh out loud. 'Estate agents are such liars. You'll never sell this place if you lie.' I walk out and shove the information she has sent me under the windscreen wipers of her car, hoping that the rain will disperse it into annoying sticky blobs. And worse.

I am evil.
No, but I am.
I must go see a man about the devil.

CHAPTER TWENTY-ONE

Holy, Sound, and Analytical Help

I sit in front of the priest, who sits in a wheelchair. His health has deteriorated since the last time I saw him but his spirit is as strong and keen as it always was. The room is full of a deep silence, born of many hours' devotion. He closes his eyes. I close mine. My thoughts jump and juggle for precedence. If only I weren't so tired I might be able to muster the energy to withdraw from them. My breathing gradually slows. Like a child, I open my eyes to get a glimpse of him. His are still closed. His head is to one side, as if what he ponders pleasantly intrigues him. His mouth is lifted at the corners as if the next thing he might do is smile. At the end of the silence he says, 'You are exactly where you need to be.' It is shocking because it goes right to the heart of my dilemma. 'Your truth is authentic. Suffering does that.' Again the silence of the room envelops us. 'Few lead authentic lives.'

Unplanned, I answer my own question: 'Why do I hate people so?' This sits on the air for a moment. 'I hate people—when I feel so ill.'

Again he goes directly to the heart of it: 'Well, it's something to have grasped that.' Suddenly I have an image of a sick animal snapping at people's heels as they pass by, uncaring and too near. That is what I was. Am. A sick animal. Hounded by the healthy. A pack sniffing out the sickly one.

The other troublesome issue that irks me makes itself felt. 'I feel so betrayed. I never knew that betrayal by a friend is the worst . . .'

He nods sagely, and gives me a direct, strong look, which makes me understand the words he has not spoken. Again we are silent. He does not mention my mother's spirit. No more do I.

I feel as if I have shed a great load. I want to give him something. I run through the Gerard Manley Hopkins poem silently in my head to check, yet again, that the words haven't deserted me. When I arrive at the end of it I am too slow to understand why he smiles and nods. It's only when I get to the end of speaking it that I am aware there was no need to have spoken it at all. He heard the silent version, which, of course, was the better of the two. As I go to leave he says, 'You have done me a power of good.' Again, I don't know whether he is speaking for him or for me. But I do when he says, 'Be gentle with them.'

The bus is full of very noisy schoolchildren. There is a girl on the right, sprawled all over an empty seat. 'Move your legs,' I say to her, in my best bossy-mother mode.

'Say please,' she taunts.

I want to scream at her, 'You shouldn't have your legs on the damn seat in the first place.'

I sit down and battle with myself for the rest of the journey, about whether I should remonstrate again with her. I keep silent. I must be getting better. Judith, the healer, although she wouldn't call herself that, welcomes me into her hallway with the most enormous hug. She is wearing a deep rich purple shirt. The colour swoops out at me. She is bright and chatty as we ascend the carpeted stairway to her small room at the back of the house. I have attended several of her workshops so her way of working is not alien to me. I trust her implicitly. All the work that I have seen her do is for the benefit and betterment of others. By their fruits . . .

'You've pulled all your energy up into your head to try to understand what you're in. Let's get some of that back into your body.' I sit on the bed and she climbs up and sits behind me, cradling me between her legs. There is something very fundamental about the way her body encases mine. Quietly from behind me comes the gentlest of gurgles that turns into a whine and a moan. It is the sound of something being born. I understand it completely. I also ache with relief at being touched. My body, even now, remembers all the weeks of being hauled about like a slab of meat. I cried out this woman's name during one of the worst times in Intensive Care. I can't remember whether it was day or night. It felt like the middle of the night, my sense of desolation was so strong. I was convinced she would hear. She would hear, but not with her ears. The moans swoop and lift. There is something awesome and of a great grandeur about these sounds, these sounds that I cannot, or have not, made for myself. These barely voiced yelps of pain are primeval. As the howls subside into a gentle, almost unvoiced delight, I feel wounds close and heal.

She lays me down carefully on the bed and places her hands on my solar plexus. I feel a rush of warmth and energy to the spot, an awareness of that part of my body, which up till now has felt vacant. It simply had not been a part of me. I learn about the vibrations of different colours and their various healing properties, and the energy to be gained from starlight. 'Odd. I bought a key-ring for myself at Christmas that had a tube of water filled with stars and moons that floated in it. Didn't realise how near to them I was about to go.' She snorts with laughter. 'I bought packets of the things from the Planetarium one morning when I walked from after seeing Dr Lewith who gave me more homeopathic drops and pills, as we swapped our new Jewish jokes. I've scattered them all over the kitchen table and stuck some on my study door so I can see them when I have my afternoon rest.'

Judith puts her hand on exactly the place in my chest where the rawness starts, my upper sternum. 'There's a chakra point here, between the throat and the heart. Its colour is turquoise.'

On my way home I buy a turquoise shawl, and some turquoise writing cards. I wrap the shawl around me instantly, and wear it for days on end. I send her a card saying, 'My body and I thank you for the afternoon and the new lease of life.'

She writes back almost immediately, saying, 'Keep the colour for yourself, you twerp.' So I go out and buy a turquoise pullover, feeling not at all guilty about spending the money for once. Everywhere I go now, I see turquoise.

I ask the girl standing next to me at the coffee van in the station if she will pass me a spoon from a pot that is further down the counter. She doesn't respond. It might be, I think, that I have spoken too quietly against the loud background noise from the station, so I say it again. There is an if-it's-not-too-much-trouble implicit in what I've said, because I suspect that's the truth. She looks at me and says, very aggressively, 'Get it yourself.' My eyes fill with tears. I find it hard to swallow the coffee. Not that much better, then.

The WOW (Wise Old Woman) says, 'Both lions belong to you. He's still the king, even though he's careworn,' and she smiles. We talk of other dreams, as Jungian analysts can often derive important information from the psyche this way, although they would be the first to admit that the dreamer's perception is the one that counts. In my eyes they stubbornly remain father and daughter. They are not mother and son.

My son remains a constant source of anger and grief. The WOW says, 'Perhaps he felt helpless?'

It's something I've not considered. The new me isn't prepared to make allowances for other people: after all, I'm the one who was—is—ill. I'm not always, hardly ever now, well enough to be able to make the extra effort to give. It's sometimes a struggle just to get through the day. To get through the humdrum business of living: shop, pay bills, post letters, do washing. She suggests that perhaps I could break away without breaking off. If I think of this as a way of protecting myself from more pain, that feels fine, but if I allow myself to dwell on him being the only family I have, I feel dumped.

302

'And after all,' says Renata quietly, 'you were dumped by your mother.'

This equation resonates all the way down my fifty-six years. It fails, however, to silence me. 'I feel I have rights now, rights to express my view, my anger. I am right because I've suffered a lot.' She says nothing.

'Is there something practical he could do?' she asks, after a moment. 'Perhaps he just doesn't know *what* to do to help?'

I don't buy that, and the anger starts to bubble more.

'It's a good warm feeling, isn't it?'

I am weary of it. Weary and frightened. But at least it shows I'm alive and kicking. Especially kicking. 'He could water the garden!' I yelp, with delight, as if landing on some miraculous, earth-shattering idea. Renata smiles and nods.

We go back over the subject of Dr X. It still rankles badly. I wrote her a letter. I recite it for Renata's entertainment: ' "Depression is a symptom of brain surgery. You added to my depression by stopping my sickness benefit. You played by the rules. We had the chance of a real friendship, but you got frightened when you said, 'I'm losing my grip.' I gave you my ex-husband's number, which cost me a lot too—I had to write to him specially. You treated me like 'one of the herd'. You're scared of establishing real relationships with your patients. And by the way—you're fired." '

That feels good. I laugh, triumphant.

Renata says soberly, 'She behaved very unsympathetically.' I feel vitiated by her judgement.

The letter doesn't get sent.

'I don't know whether I'm in strident animus mode, or whether it's a symptom of the illness. Whether the child was a broken-off bit that now is part of me . . . Round and round I go.'

'It's as if you think you are being punished by God or your mother or someone,' Renata says, interrupting my thought circles and going straight to the heart of the matter. 'As if it's your fault.'

'Well . . . Yes, I do.'

'Did the doctor say that?'

'No. He categorically said, "No," but it made no difference. It makes no difference that I still hear my foster-mother saying, "You brought it on yourself," of any childhood mishap I had. So I'm like I always was—only more so.'

'Only time will tell.'

That's the one thing I have a lot of. Time. And anger.

'Is the middle cerebral artery the emotional centre?'

I have no answer to that question.

'The brain will settle to its pre-morbid level,'

says Dr Miotto.

'That sounds grim!'

'Yes, doesn't it?' She laughs.

'I hug furry animals, I have no objectivity in front of people, I say exactly what I think. I have no tact. I sound like a child sometimes. I am at the mercy of whatever I feel.'

'Disinhibition.'

'What?'

'Disinhibition.'

I have to take a few moments to think about that. Inhibition is easy to understand. No one can afford to be inhibited in the theatre. But disinhibition. That one word ties up the myriad dreadful experiences I've had 'out in the world'.

Disinhibition.

Like myself, only more so. Impulsive. Impetuous. Blunt. Strident. Impatient. Vulnerable. Volatile.

Yes, that's a pretty morbid list.

Well, I suppose I have to be grateful that I didn't run amok up Putney High Street showing my knickers. Or worse.

'The more intelligent you are, the more understanding and insights you have and the more resources you can call on to deal with it.'

I think, Well, dealing with it's not a very accurate description of my behaviour recently, but before I can voice my thoughts she says, 'Would you like some feedback from your tests?' Oh, the tests. Of course I hadn't forgotten. Inwardly I gulp.

'The objective of the tests was to find out if there are practical deficits. It's an assessment of your cognitive functions. The last ability to go down in Alzheimer's . . .'

Oh, God, I've got Alzheimer's, I think.

'. . . for example, is the ability to read.' She flips through some more papers. 'You are at a superior level, in the top five per cent of the population. You achieved ninety-seven per cent in your intellectual functions.'

I'm already worried about the missing three per cent.

'You are under-functioning in non-verbal issues, and you are slow at information-processing, but that's typical of SAH patients. Your motor speeds—crossing out, etcetera— are OK-ish, but suggest that under pressure you find it difficult to be accurate.'

We *had*, of course, been working for one and a half hours by then. 'Damage to the frontal functions of the brain—don't let anyone hear me call it ego—means that you easily lose track of what you're doing, or of how much you've done.'

Release such as I have rarely known washes through me.

'There is no evidence of memory impairment.' The second wave is even greater than the first. I think I'm going to explode with joy. I can learn lines. I can retain those lines. Official.

'But we have to monitor the work activity. We have to learn to balance the rest and work periods.'

Me, rest? I want to go and climb a mountain and shout and sing till I'm hoarse.

'Your anxiety levels are high . . .'

Me, anxious? I don't know the meaning of the word. Not now.

'. . . which, again, is quite normal for SAHs. We'll think about you going back to work in about six months from now. We'll make a four-point plan. We'll have a session every two weeks of an hour each. Four sessions in all, and in the fourth session we'll review the situation.'

The numbers don't add up. They never did. It doesn't matter. Not now.

'All that intelligence I'm supposed to have,' I tap my head, 'that proves they put back someone else's brain.'

As I leave, I tell Dr Miotto that I'm dreading getting home on the tube. She says she finds London crowds aggressive. I say I find them torture, but an extraordinary thing happens as I get to the station. As people start passing me in ever-increasing numbers, getting on trains, going down stairs, running along corridors, all these movements that still bewilder and unsettle my balance, I can now read the degree of loss of equilibrium, both physical and mental, to be equal to the degree that my brain is tired. It is a physical symptom, not a psychological one. I Am Not Mad. But it's only now that I say that that I can allow myself to see I Have Been Mad, if mad means detached or disconnected from what the majority of people call reality. As children are. In fact, I realise my brain isn't quite a year old yet. No wonder I'm impulsive, impatient, demanding, all me-me-me as children are. I can hug my animals with impunity. I have someone on my side who knows that just getting through an ordinary day is hard. And, at last, I feel almost safe. Safe from the unpredictable. Safe from my own mind. I have someone in there with me, helping.

My bad temper, however, doesn't disappear overnight. A friend who can see the change in me that Dr Miotto's support has made confides, 'How do you think *we* felt seeing someone we love so ill?'

Immediately I think, I couldn't give a shit what you guys felt. How could I think of *you*? I was too busy battling just to get through the day.

She goes on, 'My husband thinks you don't know how ill you've been.'

I want to scream, 'Well, of course I don't! It's the thing I *think* with that's been ill.' I don't say either of these things. A small step forward. But I've never been known for keeping my mouth shut . . .

As a celebration of the test results I get into a cab, and I can feel animosity coming off the driver. Is it my voice? Is it where I'm going? He's surly, offhand, and waves of unpleasantness are coming from the driving seat.

'What are you pissed off about?' I say, giving him a chance to include me or whatever I've said in the pissed-offness.

'That's between me and the gatepost,' he says, with not an iota less attitude.

Rushing in with the best of them, I say, 'Well, please don't take it out on me. I've recently had brain surgery—'

'I'm not takin' it out on you. I'm about to have brain surgery too.'

Poor sod, I think. I flood with concern for him. Soberly I say, 'I wish you well in your brain surgery. I wish you very well.' He has no idea of the long path he faces—if there is a path for him at all.

'It was a figger of speech,' he says. I am inane.

As I open the door I hit my head. He says, 'Mind you don't hit your head, love,' and turns as I leave to say, in the kindest of voices, 'I wish you well, darlin', I really do.' It's only a small incident but it gives me hope. Somehow I have managed to turn about a potentially deeply unpleasant situation, provoked by my lack of tact. I walk along the road lightheaded, but I hear myself saying, 'How long will this last?'

During my next session Dr Miotto says, 'Intelligence and feeling are very closely linked.' I know she doesn't like talking in abstracts like this, but appreciate that she's doing it for my benefit. Neuro-psychology is, after all, a science. Cognitive therapy is about dealing with things in a practical manner. I am beginning to want to do something concrete to help myself. I need to *do*.

'The brain is the commander of everything. When we destroy the brain we destroy the basic tools of human interaction.' I nod vehemently. 'You have to learn to store your energy. We want to reach a plateau, a place where you have levelled out and feel stable, so we will break down your activities into small bits and you will chart everything you do, including your rest periods.'

This'll be a first, I think. 'Stable? What's that? How will I know when I feel it? I don't know what it feels like.'

'Well, you know, normal.'

'What's normal?' We both laugh.

How do I tell this young woman what fifteen years of being a single parent feels like? The hamster-wheel of shop, cook, clean, work, child, child, work, clean, cook, shop. Any theatre performer knows the poleaxing exhaustion of eight performances a week. Or the opposite, the gut-grinding worry of being unemployed and the accompanying how-do-I-pay-the-bills refrain.

'Has every brain patient been guilty of overwork, as I have?'

'No. It's too difficult to draw those kinds of conclusions. People's aneurysms burst for all sorts of different reasons. Smoking,' (used to be guilty), 'drinking,' (guilty), 'high blood pressure,' (not guilty), 'middle age,' (guilty), 'a blow to the head,' (low kitchen beam, guilty), 'car accidents,' (two). 'Do you overwork? Well, we'll see from your charts, won't we?' A threat is inherent somewhere. All theatre work is overwork.

Charts. Pen and paper. Great. I feel that at last I am going to do something practical to help myself and it feels terrific.

As I leave Dr Miotto hands me several sheets of information that she has taken off the Internet about ME. I am overjoyed, read it avidly. So many of the symptoms of brain surgery are the same as for ME: 'Lesions in the brain of 80% of ME patients tested . . . brain inflammation. Correlation between the areas involved and the symptoms experienced. The fatigue is not due to lack of motivation or effort.'

No, indeed. I want to *get on*. I'm estranged from the world I know. The world whose

311

language I speak. I want to *get back* into that world too.

'Lifestyle change is the foundation for recovery. ME is cyclical. How you manage your cycles is of great importance. Waking up to one of those precious "good days" is like finding £100 in your pocket.' I'll say. 'You want to make up for lost time. You want to go out and spend it all. You want to do everything you've been deprived of. This is a rare opportunity to get a lot done.' Indeed. So I do. Only more so. It says *'Don't'*.

Nevertheless, the following morning I begin to have the second good day that I have had in a year. The next day is good too, the third. I am euphoric. I am also very stupid. I think, I'm through it. It's over. I'm well. Then I crash. Back to square one.

Along with the other clichés I've collected on this journey, 'Don't overdo it,' 'You were in the right place at the right time,' I now hear, 'Two steps forward and one back,' although it feels far from that ratio.

'You can use the good day to help build momentum towards healing. Think of the good day as a form of capital that can be invested in your healing process, rather than being spent or squandered. On a good day make a list of all that you feel you can do. Do *half* the things on your list then *stop*. For the next day or two observe your body's responses. If you crash, your assessment is adjusted

312

downwards on your next good day.' What, me? I never do things by halves.

Of course, as I proceed with the charts, the tangible evidence of what I do is so condemnatory in its busyness that I have to begin to *make* time to put my feet up—or, rather, my back down on the sitting-room floor, just to show Dr Miotto that I have taken on board what she says. I am forced to rest. Her first glance at my doings makes her gasp. I am sent away to try harder not to try hard. That's all part of it, I'm sure. But it is hard. The minutes tick by so slowly, and what feels like an hour of watching the ceiling—or, in the cottage, the cobwebs on the ceiling—is usually almost exactly a miserly twenty minutes. Twenty minutes of doing nothing but hearing my brain chatter, prattle, squawk and whine. However much I rest, however early I go to bed—to read mostly (I'm now up to my fifty-eighth book this year), however many nutritious meals I eat, I don't feel any better at all. It is very dispiriting. But Dr Miotto is there. When anything happens to me that I can't deal with or understand, it goes into the notebook for discussing at the next session. My life becomes a desert of time in between sessions, and an oasis of comfort during one. I know about the danger of becoming dependent on a therapist. I'm utterly, pathetically dependent on Dr Miotto, but I don't care a jot. What's more, she's suggested that my son come to a session so that at last I stand to have an ally, once it's understood that my particular form of crankiness isn't particular to me but general to most brain patients. Happy to be of the herd.

I've had my driving licence back for a couple of months, but it's only now that I feel I might just be able to manage driving—only down a few country lanes, of course. The local garage comes and tows away my ancient car to check it out—especially the tyres, which it has sat on for nearly twelve months—and to give it an MOT. I am very nervous indeed about driving again and enlist a friend who lives opposite to come with me. Supposing I lose my concentration? Forget where I am? Not notice a red light? I am now very aware of losing track of what I am doing when I'm tired, and I am tired all the time. The more I think about it, the more terrifying a prospect it becomes. He promises to take over the wheel if it all becomes too much for me. As I reverse out, my neck and head whine and zap, and a stiletto of pain stabs me behind the right eye. I flinch, but go on after his encouragement to get out on to the road.

I feel as if I have never driven in my life. Every car that comes out from a side turning makes me jump. Every T-junction is a test of nerves. I'd driven for over thirty years, and it had become an automatic series of actions with involuntary responses. Not any more. I can't trust this new self. Every turn of the head, every look is a decision that has to be made consciously It is exhausting. After ten minutes he says he thinks that's enough for one day.

He is right. When we arrive home I can barely muster the energy to lift up my legs, put them down on the ground and stand up to get out of the car. He has to help lift me out and I have to lean on him to get to the back door. His beard brushes my cheek. I start, and almost send his glasses flying. We look at the car and smile. Another tangle with the 'real world' completed. Another step towards being independent.

Someone wants to buy my house. I can't believe it. I also can't allow myself to acknowledge the tremor of fear this brings. At last I've sold the house. Action stations. Go to measure up the flat (I last saw—if it's still free) for curtains and make a list of what I need. Enlist another opinion. Get son to come with me to view it through his eyes. It's a practical task, after all, and our difficult patch seems to have been levelled out into a working relationship that's been improved by the practical task of his watering the pots in my garden several times since I first broached the idea. He likes the flat. I like the flat even more.

What will I do with all my books? he asks. Where will I put all my clothes? There are no shelves of any serviceable size, and the wardrobe is a built-in job for people who haven't hoarded much-loved clothes for twenty years, as I have. Why does he keep bringing up problems? It notches up my frustration levels. I start sentences that trail off in mid-air as I write. I used to be able to write as I talked, but now it seems beyond me. I either say the word I'm writing, or write the word I'm saying. It worries and confuses me. The list is a nonsense of words I've said, not things I need. I start the list yet again. As we walk back along the bridge, my words start to slip and slide. It takes such a lot of energy to talk while walking. I try to gloss over it, but he has seen me notice that he noticed the slurring. Darleney has promised she will help with the move if she's not working. Cherry too. My son adds exactly the same proviso. I envisage moving day with all three of them otherwise employed, and the back of my throat smarts. 'It's what it will do to your health, Ma,' he says, rather sheepishly. I am livid with him for finding such stupid excuses to blight the plans for my new life, and it's only the numbing effect of the first half of a glass of wine that stops me storming out of the pub.

I find out that the man who wants to buy my house is a property developer. I am outraged. This is not right. This is a home. It must stay a home. I can see that my estate agent has also joined the swelling ranks of those who think I am insane.

On an escalator to get yet another train back to the country, a man bumps into my little suitcase on wheels with his briefcase, ripping a catch off it in the process. 'Don't knock me over! I've been ill!' I shout, after his retreating back. Uselessly I try to stick the catch back into the gaping holes. I sound like a cranky old lady. Now I'm sane enough to understand that I do sound mad.

My son doesn't come to the next session after all. Dr Miotto and I wait and wait. I have been so eager that he should be informed. Even if he can't make allowances for me, at least he will know my crankiness is a physical state and when I'm tired to give me a wide berth. Then he won't fall prey to the general destruction of everything that occurs around me and within me when I'm in that state of utter exhaustion. He rings eventually in response to one of the many calls Dr Miotto has made to say that he's taking care of a girlfriend who's in hospital. I am heartbroken. I sob with disappointment like the child I revert to when tired. After we've mopped me up, we start the session and Dr Miotto tells me she is going back to Brazil. For good. Soon. In two weeks. I feel bereft, abandoned, rejected, dejected and in despair. I spend most of the session in tears. Square one, here I am again. I don't listen to anything she says, particularly not the bits where she emphasises that all these tears indicate that I have been Doing Too Much. She talks about another neuro-psychologist she knows who is doing the same sort of work. I listen half-heartedly. I know I am not being reasonable but I also know it won't be the same.

Christmas approaches, the Christmas I nearly didn't see. It is inexplicably significant. I cook Christmas Eve and Christmas Day dinner for Darlene and Ken. I am happy to be cooking again. Friends plan to throw a party to celebrate my having survived a year. I am happy. I celebrate meeting the man with a beard and glasses who, as in the dream I had in Intensive Care, *does* live next to a church. His house is crammed with books. He is also a Leo. Now I know why I was drawn back to this village after twenty-five years. He lives opposite. In more ways than one it seems dreams are portents.

CHAPTER TWENTY-TWO

Brain-Life-Buoy

It seems odd to be travelling in the opposite direction for a neuro-psychology session. Even odder that in just another week it will be a year to the day that I collapsed. A year. An absurd amount of time. On bad days I feel I have made no progress whatsoever. Friends hug me at the party and say how well I've done, but I don't believe them. I don't seem to have done anything. I make jokes about having very good but very *tired* guardian angels. My wish to get back to work in the theatre seems as far away as it ever did. I am just as impatient, impulsive and bad-tempered. Sleep, or lack of it even with drugs, is still a problem, as are headaches, which still can obliterate me for three to four days on end.

My bearded one becomes a dab hand at juggling ice-packs for neck and head, and musters endless, inordinate amounts of patience. It helps that I now really do have an ally. Someone who can see my eyes 'drop out with tiredness', my face 'grow grim and grey', long before I am willing to admit or sometimes even know I am in trouble. He learns to recognise all sorts of signs. This companionship and care is beyond comfort. It is balm to the

319

soul. It is also a huge turning point. I feel very lucky. Wretched but lucky and loved.

My son calls him the Godsend. My friend John P calls him Nerves of Steel.

Then I meet Dr Baehr and the balance is tipped even more in favour of good fortune. She is a statuesque, softly spoken, blonde American, which endears me to her as soon as she opens her mouth. I have no idea at the time how important this doctor is going to become in my life. I am still mourning the loss of Dr Miotto, the loss of my work, the loss of several friends, the loss of the world I knew, and the loss of confidence and trust in myself. She is, unknown to me, going to teach me how to live again. This is the woman who, patiently and quietly over the next year, and then some, as all neuro-psychologists do, really gives me the tools to handle my new life.

I blurt and burble and prattle out the last year in no chronological order. Words tumble over each other, slur and jar and slide out of my control. I suppose if there is an order in it at all, it's in degrees of hurt. Son, job, friends, health. Several times she tells me to take deep breaths. I do. Then off I charge again. She doesn't interrupt. She doesn't castigate. She refers, from time to time, to the papers I assume have come from Mr Kitchen and Mr Y.

Time eludes me. I worry about it. I must have talked my way through the entire first session and out the other side. She says, 'I have an agenda to help you with what you need, not what time it is. That's why I don't wear a watch.'

I have trouble believing things can be this good.

'Any blood spill in the brain causes the brain to swell slightly. It hits the hard skull, compresses, and one of the results is major fatigue, decreased concentration and slowed mental speed. It usually takes a year for neural stability to be achieved. Until then it will interfere with your concentration, and you may well be irritable and tearful at times. Your friends will expect you to behave as you always did because you look the same.'

I am so aghast at the accuracy of this that I don't know whether to scribble it in my ever-present notebook or just bathe in the solace of her words.

'You are still at risk. You have a lot more living to do. We will start with stabilising your schedule. A regular bedtime.'

'The regular bedtime for a working theatre actor is about one a.m.'

She avoids the obvious, but I hear in my head: 'You are no longer a working theatre actor.'

But Dr Baehr just says, even more gently, 'It won't be your bedtime for ever, but for now, yes. We are trying to help the body recover. You have a two-fold crisis to manage. The emotional shock, the trauma of being so near death and the physical side of being in Intensive Care that long, plus the insult to the brain that clipping an aneurysm causes. Your state is a medical fact.'

She is giving me the right to feel all right about feeling awful. Immediately half of the rock between my shoulders melts away.

'Keep dangerous thoughts at bay, they are a medical fact. We must get you to level off at a stage (irony) of improvement, or you will continue, as you are, on a roller-coaster of feeling good, then crashing. It's like dieting, then bingeing. All or nothing.'

All those images are shamingly familiar. Blessed are they that heal, I think. Even more blessed are they that heal the wounds that can't be seen.

I say those exact words seven months later when I'm opening the new wing of the hospital where she has been treating me. It's another good test. To speak in public, but my own words this time. Not many patients can have had that kind of privilege. That day Dr Baehr introduces me to some more of her patients, two of them considerably younger than me, both in wheelchairs. During the next few months I'm going to witness the Lebanese girl, who is now semi-comatose with an arm in plaster, shed the wheelchair and manage several triumphant steps with a walking frame.

The other group, standing a way apart,

greet me with, 'Hi. Hi. Hi. We're divas too.'

'Oh?' I wonder out loud. 'Are you dancers or musicians?'

'No. I'm an investment banker. She's a broker in the City.'

The dig stings. Then, Oh, of course, I think, this is private medicine. Hence the high-powered jobs.

'*She* fell off a horse. *This one* hit her head on a table. She had a stroke,' pointing to a willowy, tawny-skinned beauty of no more than thirty with huge almond-shaped eyes. A bond is formed between us all. We have all been in varying kinds of the same boat.

'Are you Spanish?'

'Yes.'

'Oh, how awful for you to be taken ill in a strange country. So far from home.'

Her eyes fill with tears. What a crass sod I am. I put my arm round her.

'No. No,' she says, mopping at her face. 'I had my mother with me.'

'Oh, what a worry for her, but how lovely,' I say, 'to have the best person in the world look after you.' I am full of envy.

'I couldn't wait for her to go back to Spain,' she snuffles, 'she was driving me mad.'

'Don't you get on?'

'Yes, yes, we're very close. But she didn't understand what had happened to me.'

'You look the same but behave different,' we chorus, almost in unison.

The horse lady turns to me and says brusquely, 'Who are you, anyway? I've never heard of you. What films have you been in? What TV have you done? I've never seen you.'

I am knocked off my precarious balance by her bluntness. My confidence in shreds, I manage—probably only because Dr Baehr is within reach, should I sink under this onslaught: 'Hang on a minute. Hang on. I'm a brain patient too. I can't take much of this.' Speaking in public was a double whammy. It has leeched the few wisps of energy I did have. All gone in the wave of adrenaline.

'Well, I'm sorry but I just have to say the truth. I just have to. I have to say the truth.' I motion for her to let up. It's coming at me in huge waves. I am being bludgeoned, overwhelmed, rubbed up the wrong way, walked over. Here I am, face to face with my own symptoms.

Between us, Dr Baehr and I develop a more intricate timetable than the one I had with Dr Miotto, which was simply accounting for each hour:

9 a.m.	morning pages/quiet time/mail
11	shower/wash hair
12–1.30	shop, high street lunch
2	read and [sometimes] rest
3–4–5	tidy house/potter in garden
6	phone calls/supper

8.30	bed early/read more
10	wake up/read more
2 a.m.	wake up/read more

The truth of the agenda is rather different.

'Quiet Time' brings me face to face with how my body hurts and how incapable I still am of anything resembling meditation, my mind darting all over the place and taking my attention with it—usually down avenues that lead to negativity and depression, no work, no money, etc. I often have to leave my meditation chair because I cannot bear any more tears.

'Mail': I panic over nasty letters—usually from the private health-insurance people, who are arguing over a claim for acupuncture (£70) or osteopathy or some similar treatment (£30) that keeps my neck or back at least at a manageable level of pain. (This is the same company that didn't have to pay £21,000 plus for my treatment in Intensive Care as the agreement between all the EU countries (Form E1–11) paid for that.) This private health-care scheme is chaotic in its system of paying refunds (when they *are* eventually paid) it doesn't actually inform me as to which of the £30-worth of medical bills is being refunded. So I am frequently owed two or three hundred pounds, which I can ill afford. Liable as my brain is to going round in spirals over figures or dates, I am frequently reduced to shouting down the phone at this organisation, which purports to an interest in health care. At least I have the comfort, on one memorably rare occasion, of a sympathetic listener from Customer Services at the other end of the phone for a change. The next day I am the recipient of an extravagant bunch of rich pink gerberas and roses, complete with a card of apology for the stress they have caused me. So, I am not going mad. They were incompetent. It wasn't me. The following day another identical bunch arrives, complete with card, an exact replica of the first. I look at the twin bunches at opposite ends of the sitting room and worry about my grasp on reality.

The pension people, too, are a regular source of *Angst*. They want another list of hours worked. They have already diminished their payment to me during the time I taught for BADA at Balliol so I live in daily terror that this regular little income is going to be reduced yet again. Ironic that the two private health-care factors in my life cause me (and will go on causing me) more stress than almost anything else. Dr Baehr suggests she writes to them to let them know how I'm getting on. I want to fall prostrate at her feet with gratitude.

'Shop, high street' scores maximum points on the frustration scale. I am always too tired to do it. There are always too many people in the street. The ones who pass quickly unbalance me. The ones who move slowly get in my way. The queue I am in is always too slow. I push people out of the way. I mutter curses under my breath at people who come too close. I fume and rage at something I can't get, no matter how many shops I try. Shopping becomes synonymous with biting people's heads off. Dr Baehr suggests I list these incidents as part of the cognitive therapy. I decide to call them HBOs. Heads Bitten Off. There is something palliative about the act of writing them down, as if seeing them on the page goes some way to removing the sting. I still hate the world with a healthy appetite, though, and have now, thanks to this list, tangible evidence that it certainly hates me.

On one journey, a bus conductor, female, with Frida Kahlo eyebrows that didn't need the help from the eyebrow pencil they so lavishly got, vivid scarlet lips and a wiry candyfloss of black-dyed hair, tells me to sit down in no uncertain terms and an undeniable Belfast accent as I attempt to hold on to the upright rail in the bus to diminish the amount I'm lurching. I have already taken exception to the way she looks and explain that I have to stand up before the bus gets to the stop as I've had brain surgery and need time to adjust to the upright position. 'Sit down or you'll fall,' she says dismissively. Of course she's right, but I go on being thrown from side to side, my arm wrenched this way and that, as the bus heaves its way round a corner. Pig-headed, me, but more so.

'Tidy house and potter in garden' is a euphemism for fretting about why my cleaning lady, who I thought was a friend, should leave now when I need her most. Endless hours of worry there. Worry plus guilt, too, about having all this space empty and gathering dust while I am in the country, and a loathing for how banal and domestic my life has become, my escape route into the theatre still blocked. A play is so all-absorbing, all-demanding: rehearsals insist that real life should be put on hold. Humankind cannot bear much housewifery.

I go to the second dream flat with another friend, Pat, this time on a Saturday morning, to measure up for curtains. Pop music is blaring from the flat above, and I can hear a small child running up and down and round and round on wooden floors. Pat O and I stare at each other, speechless. What an ideal noise mixture for getting over brain damage. While I insist on finding out via the solicitor which of the tenants actually *owns* the flats they live in, and why the carpeting-everywhere rule is being broken by 'them upstairs', the owner of the second dream flat sells it to someone else. So I'm back to square one again, except this time I have a buyer interested in my home but nowhere to move to. The London house sits round my neck like an albatross. It's too much for me to take care of alone: a little light dusting has a way of turning into major heaving of furniture and obsessive spring-cleaning of room after room till I wonder why my back aches and my eyes smart and itch from the polish. Losing track, oh, yes.

I read and read to stop me thinking. Occasionally I wake to find my specs still on and my book under my hand, but these occasions are rare. The more I read the more my brain wakes up. Although I have actually, for the first time in my adult life, begun to detect when I go through the sleep-imminent barrier into more wakefulness. Layer upon layer of years of fatigue is being slowly undone. Perversely I often think, Read on, it's one of the few pleasure you have. I have indulged it to the full. The book count at the end of the year is fifty-eight.

Dr Baehr is horrified. 'Try to rest for the same amount of time you read.'

'Rest for three hours? Not possible, Dr Baehr.'

A wry smile. 'Read for only half an hour then . . .'

I was always a bookworm. As a child, books were my escape from the war between my mother and my foster-mother. Or my foster-mother telling me how bad my mother was to have had me. Pregnant at nineteen. And a war on.

Then there's clothes shopping. 'Why am I obsessed with clothes? Is it because I have to find a new look for this new body of mine?'

Dr Baehr says, 'It may be because shopping is the only social interaction you have now.'

'Oh.'

Cognitive therapy is like that.

Actually, my bum's got so fat none of my trousers fit. Also, the memory of my mother's scorn on the cheaply dressed child from England still rankles.

'We all need structure in our lives. You are an achiever. Shopping makes you feel you've accomplished something.'

That it should come to this.

I make a stand for the importance of symbolism, archetypes, dreams and spirituality. Dr Baehr says, 'You can come back to all that after. All the spiritual and philosophical aspects will still be there for you. It's not what we're dealing with here.'

No more it isn't.

Apart from my HBO list, I am then engaged in a more detailed chart of action in relation to feeling. The actions are listed according to the energy they take from me and the feelings are listed in order of degrees of stress and pain:

Key of activity
10 Teaching/working
9 Tube/crowds/travelling
8 Shopping
7 Housework/mail
6 Cooking/gardening

330

5 Sitting
4 Writing/walking
3 Reading
2 Meditating/resting
1 Sleeping

Key of feeling
10 Tears/despair/depression
9 Raw chest/back pains
8 Very tired
7 Not OK
6 Just OK (difficult to define)
5 OK
4 Well
3 Up and able
2 Fine
1 Really well

In both columns 5 is a kind of stable 'norm'. The day is divided into four sections: a.m., noon, p.m., and night. One of the objectives is to keep the daily score below twenty-five in each column. Often at the beginning, if I go over twenty-five in the activity column I end up for the next few days with the 8s, 9s and 10s in the feeling column.

I enjoy writing and walking. Although they are absorbing and demand concentration, I feel they don't use up as much energy as cooking or gardening. With the latter it's easier to drift from one thing to another without realising it. The key of feeling is

331

harder to assess. Often I can go from 5 to 8 in a flash. It is possible to have, for example, 3 and 8, or 10 and 5 (9 and 5 is a rarity). The other point of this chart, and the one I invent myself—which has date?/state?/exercise?/pills/rest?/and hours slept?—is not just to see how the individual day has gone in terms of my state of mind and the amount of energy, and pills, used, but to see if a pattern develops over a length of time. It does. It is also an alarmingly accurate record of peaks and troughs. Many times Dr Baehr shakes her head slowly and quietly while studying my charts, and repeats, 'We must stabilise your schedule. You are still at risk.'

I catch sight of one of the other patients' charts. In the activity column, it has 'socialising' and 'gym'. I realise what a hermit I've become, apart from the odd half-day of teaching. A happy hermit. Listening to music on the radio, knitting by the fire with the Godsend. Thrills and spills. 'Gym' puts my infrequent dawdles up the hill into the right perspective. I whine about this to Dr Baehr. 'I couldn't get to the gym, let alone function inside it.'

'No two head injuries are the same. No two recoveries are the same. People are ignorant of the timescale of brain convalescence.'

I'll say. Me too. I make a new promise to myself to manage the overreach of my spirit, so that my poor old body gets a chance to recover. This is a serious notion. Not like learning the piano, or walking the Andes.

'I feel dreadful. I am overtired. I am ashamed of overworking. Three half-mornings of teaching—I really enjoyed it, but it takes days and days for the adrenaline to leave my body. Till it does, I'm caught in the same trap: headaches, painkillers, forgetting to eat—I'm so overtired I have no appetite—brain goes into overdrive, I can't sleep. I have raw pains in my chest.'

'You must try to pace yourself consistently. The half-days you work you must keep them empty of anything else. It's a professional engagement. You must be at peak performance level. Protect your work.'

This is the one time I hear a note of concern in her voice: she's worried that if I get overtired I will snap and damage my working life. This in turn worries me. I still have little ability to manage my irritation and bluntness. So I am in danger of damage.

'Make your work sacred.'

Quite.

'Your expectations can't be met by your body. These charts are a learning process. If you've got yourself to "chest pains" you've missed the earlier warning signs from your body. People can only take the roller-coaster for so long. Your body will take control of the situation again.'

Point taken. Even though it is said in a calm,

matter-of-fact way, it is driven home hard because I am still unshakeable in the belief that, in spite of all that has been said, I brought this on myself.

'Any seeds that you plant for your new life will be smashed up by the roller-coaster. You haven't even got to level ground yet. Take time. Heal. Rest. Relax. This is a chance to take stock. A golden opportunity for change.'

What she really means is, 'Get rid of those bad habits.'

'How many people have the luxury of getting off the treadmill and having a good long look at their life? A chance for reappraisal?'

'Mmm.'

'It may not feel like that now but it will.'

'A new life? Oh, yes, it does feel like a new life. That's why I'm selling my house and moving to a new flat, only I haven't got the flat bit right yet.'

'Moving?'

'Well, I hope to be.'

'Moving?'

There is no denying the implication behind that one word. I say nothing for a change.

'Moving house is very stressful and demanding. Is now the right time?'

I take my house off the market and myself out of the firing line.

Was my SAH in the limbic area of the brain?

Is every SAH patient obsessed by it?

What is the limbic area?

Am I at a different level of perception?

Has it changed my relationship to everyone?

Is my judgement impaired?

Do most people go through a personality change?

Why is it taking me so long to feel 'normal'?

I can't trust myself or my reactions—is that 'normal'?

'Why am I asking so many questions?'

'Can I ask you one? The pension company want to look at the results of your tests—is that OK?' says Dr Baehr.

'What? The MRI scans from Paris?'

'No, only a brain surgeon could understand those.'

'Mr Kitchen still has them?'

'Yes. They want the neuro-psychology tests.'

'When I came top of the class? Sure. Why hide my light under a bushel?'

She laughs and we begin another of my fortnightly life-saving sessions.

'The brain is the most sophisticated machine known to man.'

'One of the last frontiers of the unknown,' I say, pompously, and then explain, 'I bought

myself the Susan Greenfield book *Brain Story.*
I also bought *The Private Life of the Brain* and
The Brain—a Guided Tour.'

'So, you're an expert, huh?'

'Hardly. What does the middle cerebral
artery do?'

'It's very hard to say a certain part of the
brain deals only with a certain function. The
middle cerebral artery carries the brain's main
blood supply. So fresh blood was being
pumped all the time you were drifting in and
out of consciousness.'

'Was it the morphine that made me drift like
that?'

'No, you wouldn't have been given
morphine *before* the operation. They would
need to see exactly what the brain was doing.'

'But I felt no pain.' I marvel at how cleverly
the brain blanks out too much pain.

'You were unconscious.'

'And my brain was full of blood before they
operated on me?'

'Yes.'

I count on my fingers: 'Tuesday,
Wednesday, Thursday, Friday.'

'You could have had horrendous deficits.'
So I could.

I *am* lucky.

We both sit quietly, a rarity for me. I come
in here to her quiet grey office and usually give
vent to all the stuff I've been storing up,
unpack all the mishaps and hardships since the

last visit, blurt them out and blast her with them. She is never less than calm and poised. Her voice is always carefully modulated.

'I'm obsessive about losing things now. I can't allow myself to get on with anything else till I've found it.'

'All our shortcomings, our personal foibles are accentuated after brain surgery.'

That shuts me up. Impetuous. Impatient. Obsessive. Tetchy. Opinionated. Yes, that fits. And those are only the good things.

'The limbic system—to go back to one of your other questions—is the seat of the emotions.'

Well, that's obviously been damaged too. 'Has it been damaged?'

She checks some papers.

'No, it hasn't.'

'I still can't bear to have my space invaded on the tube.'

'Pace yourself. Don't travel when you're tired. We need to have you feeling balanced and stable for at least three months.'

Twelve weeks? I think I'm lucky if I have two *days* of calm a month. The charts are there to prove it. 'I still get very irritable. With myself and with the world.'

'Of course, you're now more aware of your attention span, and if you can't maintain it that, too, will make you irritable.'

'I sometimes think I'm frightened of everything. Everything scares me. I don't feel

337

I belong to the world. Sometimes . . . I wonder . . .' The tissues are offered.

'People, brain patients, get scared. Families feel helpless too. People always withdraw if they feel helpless.'

The silence hangs in the air. I realise that, in her mellifluous way, she has answered all my questions.

'Would you like your son to come to a session here?'

'Yes, oh, yes, please.' I mop up. 'Susan Greenfield says we are our brains. Our brains are what other people perceive as us. That's scary. Right now that's scary.'

'You have more potential now than you ever had.'

I think, churlishly, Don't give me all that Californian New Age stuff. 'I rest and I don't feel better.'

'Yes, that's hard. No "good-behaviour reinforcement". There's no immediate improvement, I know. It's hard. What you are doing is really hard. Patients want to hold on to the "old life"—the life they are familiar with.'

'Why?'

'Because that's what they know. There's comfort and security in it.'

'Why *am* I asking so many questions?'

'You are in a reflective mode. Before, you were in a survival mode.'

'Before? Last year?'

'The first year.'

'Survival?'

'Yes.'

Survival reminds me of death. Somewhere I read recently about the stages of grief: shock; anger; denial; loss; acceptance. Except I seem to have gone: shock; anger; denial; anger; loss; anger. Anger. Anger. Anger.

'Survival, did you say, Dr Baehr?'

'Yes.'

'And denial?'

'Yes.'

'Denial? For a whole year? I have been pretending—for a whole year—that none of this has happened?'

'Yes. From what I've seen of your part-time work charts, yes.'

Silence.

'You were in shock.'

'Well, I certainly am now.'

CHAPTER TWENTY-THREE

Heaven, Hell and Help

On the tube I catch, between the swaying bodies, from the comfort of the seat that I have asked for, glimpses of this poem which I struggle to write down:

I saw Eternity the other night
Like a great ring of pure and endless light
All calm as it was bright,
And round beneath it Time, in hours,
    days, years,
Driv'n by the spheres,
Like a vast shadow mov'd, in which the
    world
And all her train were hurl'd . . .

'A great ring of pure and endless light'
reminds me of a dream I had before I was ill,
about a great white plate, above me in the
darkness, a plate full of white food being
offered me. That, in turn, brings to mind the
white bowl full of blood-stained vomit after I
collapsed. There seems to be a symmetry in
there somewhere. These images resonate a
good while.

I visit the Wise Old Woman.

At first I am reluctant to talk about
cognitive therapy. It seems almost a betrayal of
her wisdom, her, and my respect for many
mysteries. But when I do describe Dr Baehr
and her sayings, she says simply, with a smile,
'There's more to Dr Baehr than her
professional background.'

I nod.

'Yes, you will see things differently now.
After the Night Sea Journey. Something in you
will touch people deeply because of your near-
death experience.' I feel I am the guardian of

340

something that is unknowable.

She has looked at my birth chart. 'The sun in the sixth house means you must look after your body.'

I wonder how will I answer not taking care of it now? I bought a fridge magnet in America that said, 'If you don't take care of your body where will you live?' It made me smile at the time. Now I see it as a remonstrance.

The right side of the brain is the 'female' side. So I've had a massive wake up call to the feminine. And that was *before* I met the Godsend.

'This was meant to be,' says the WOW. 'Somebody must have intervened for you to be still here.'

I receive a card from David that was sent to him by a Roman Catholic priest-friend: 'I'm saying a mass for JL's intentions on Ash Wednesday, but she's much in my prayers before that. I'm sure a saintly Tudor queen is praying for her too. I think of them linked across the centuries and I'm sure that Katharine will be keeping a grateful and watchful eye on her.'

I am deeply moved by it. I loved Katharine of Aragon.

A woman who works at my hairdresser's, Sylvie, whom I have known since we were both young enough not to have dyed hair, comes up to me quietly and says, 'I lit candles for you and prayed that you would be all right.' This is a side of her I never dreamed she had. There are several like her who tell me, in surprising places, at unexpected times, that they have prayed for me. Closet Christians.

On Tuesday 3 April a year and three months AC my son gets to a session of neuro-psychology. Dr Baehr runs it largely as educational information-giving in terms of what an aneurysm is and does when it bursts. She steers away from anything to do with mother/son relationships and gets me to suggest practical ways in which he can be of help. We are to avoid any direct discussions about what the illness did to our relationship. It's too much for me to handle, and it makes him angry. We show him all my charts. Dr Baehr is full of encouragement about how I am managing more demanding tasks and not crashing quite so often. He smiles at the HBO lists. Between us we tell the joke of my saying in Intensive Care, 'My bullshit tolerance is absolutely zero now.'

And him saying, 'It was never very high, Ma.'

Dr Baehr says 'The frontal lobe manages impulse control. We think of lots of things, but we don't necessarily say them.'

But I do. I have, for over a year.

I realise, with dread, that I have said exactly what I felt and what I thought in every situation I have been in. Small wonder I have been alone—till the Godsend turned up.

Turned up trumps.

'So, let's devise a scheme for helping those outbursts—preventing them occurring because it's not useful behaviour for your professional reputation.'

A chill in my gut accompanies my wondering what my snapping heads off may have already done. I remember the young writer of a radio play whom I told off for giving notes to the actors. 'That's the director's job,' I said, 'not yours.' The director agreed with me, but I wonder how he felt about my delineating his job. Bossy and blunt. Always was. Only more so.

'Let's use the five-point plan.' She stretches out her hand with its long fingers and red-varnished nails and ticks off the points one by one. 'One: where are you? Remind yourself you're not at home, therefore you're *not safe*. Two: leave the room. Go to the toilet—go out for a coffee. Get yourself out of the potentially explosive situation.'

'That's not always possible in a recording studio.'

'Three: what are the consequences of you saying what you're burning to say? Four: what results will that have? Or Five: walk away. Leave it alone.'

'WLCRW,' says my son, having already put it into a mnemonic for me. I feel a little cherished.

'The frontal lobe controls all initiation of

343

behaviour. Think of it as the executive secretary of the brain.'

My secretary has been sprawled flat out on her desk in a coma. 'Away from her desk' in a big way.

'So, remember, you guys, one phone call a week each. If you tell him you're exhausted, you must both end the phone call right there. If he says he can't speak right now, you ring back your mom within two hours. OK?'

We nod like the good children we want to be.

'If the conversation is escalating out of control, either one of you can say, "Time out."' She looks at me. 'You call me if you don't feel emotionally stable.' I know she knows what a huge life-buoy this is.

'And, both of you, keep the topic Recent.'

'Keep it Modern,' says my son, as if the idea is not new to him at all.

The phone rings. While she answers it, we smile nervously at each other. I have managed not to say any of the hurtful accusatory stuff that I know now has been largely responsible for driving us apart. The terror of what I have been is diminishing in the light of learning how to handle, just a little, this new person I am now.

Dr Baehr puts the phone down and adopts her extra-quiet voice and her gentle look, which means something hard to handle is about to be introduced in the most undramatic

344

fashion. 'Now, this isn't going to be a problem because I will deal with it, and give them more information about you. But that was the sickness pension company doctor. He has read your test results. As you have no impairments he thinks you should come off the pension and go back to work full-time now.'

The worst aspect of the uncontrollable shrieking is that it happens in front of my son. Just when he was beginning to feel a bit safer with me. I am aflame with the injustice of it. I love my job. The implication is that I am malingering. I am incandescent that yet another medic knows so little about the tortuous path to recovery from brain surgery. That yet another so-called 'health' company should have been the cause of such major anguish. I am shaking with distress and fighting to get my breath. I am in full panic-attack.

Dr Baehr bundles my son out of the room and me into her private toilet to wash my face and try to collect myself. I am past being able to control my breath and have to wait, gripping the washbasin, while the attack runs its course. This in itself is frightening. I am utterly out of control. I am at the mercy of yet more engulfing waves of despair. As they begin to wear themselves out my anger flickers palely and attempts to grow again, but it is a poor, shredded thing. I feel, as I have felt before, with Dr X and Mr Y, that I would have received more understanding if I had sat around being ill and done nothing. I feel as if I have been beaten with a hammer.

Dr Baehr goes to fetch my son and order me some more tea. I hear her say as they walk back into the room, 'This is very distressing to your mother as she is frightened.'

My son walks to the tube with his arm round my shoulders. I dread the moment when our journeys will divide.

It does set me back. Back, and down. Whenever I think of it I am hopping mad. I actually shift from foot to foot to manage my fury. It flares up sporadically for days after. After each eruption I feel physically as if I've been hit. The cost of the emotions of rage and fear wears me down too. Feeling wretched is a tiring burden, on top of worrying about the lack of money coming in. However, it is being harassed by an organisation into which I have paid funds for years to protect myself that really has me spitting fire. Dr Baehr is on the phone to them, fighting my patch, explaining patiently about brain fatigue, dizziness, emotional extremes, inability to handle stress. She then writes a calm, explanatory letter. I write a furious explanatory letter. I really enjoy it. I point out in carefully crafted sarcasm that I would hardly have taken my house off the market, still not be driving in London, or been unable to manage £20,000 worth of TV work if

I were well. This letter I *do* send.

Eventually my little pension is reinstated. I can breathe out again, and concentrate on getting well—until the next onslaught. The Godsend enjoys the irony of the insurance company making me feel worse and therefore prolonging my convalescence. They are provoking the very thing they wish to curtail. The humour of it isn't lost on me. I just don't have the energy to laugh. The ghastliness at least makes me take extra rest. I try not to think about it, as it presses my bomb-release button and I'm off again, ranting, wasting the invaluable minute reserves of energy I do have. So we develop a Help Tactic. A Help-I-can't-deal-with-another-syllable-more. Dr Baehr calls it a warning sign. We decide to call it *'drapeau rouge'*—DR for short. The Godsend makes me a rather medieval-looking one in red paper, on a toothpick, stuck in a cork. It is delightful. I know I will be a long way from delight, though, when I am obliged to use it. As we live in a democracy, at least as far as spitting blood when we both get overtired, I insist he makes one for himself to protect him from my rants. He urges, in Dr Baehr's words, that I 'don't go down there'. I write a large note on my desk that says, 'Don't feed the monster.' Well, I know what I mean, thanks to another tool in the cognitive-therapy battery that Dr Baehr insists, in the quietest and politest way, of course, that I use. I have

347

been introduced to *The Feel Good Book* by Dr David Burns. Awful title. Dr Baehr foresees my mockery, apologises for the Californian New Ageness of it, and insists, in her amiable, affable way, that 'It works.' One of its basic premises has me hooting with derision: 'Just because you *feel* it, it doesn't make it right.' But I've spent thirty-five years trusting what I feel. That's my job.

My profession is taught to craft the playwright's words and the character's feelings into human behaviour. How can I stop relying on my feelings?

It lists the kind of wrong-thinking that causes depression. I can stop that: it tells me how to.

(1) All or nothing: falling short of perfection is total failure.
(2) Overgeneralisation: one thing negative—it's all a never-ending pattern of defeat.
(3) Mental filter: picking out a single negative detail, dwelling on it exclusively so all becomes darkened.
(4) Disqualifying the positive: somehow good things don't count.
(5) Jumping to conclusions: make a negative decision even though there are no facts to support it.
   (a) mind-reading: assuming other people's negative reaction to you.
   (b) the fortune-teller: things will turn out badly.

(6) Catastrophising: you exaggerate the importance of things.
(7) Emotional reasoning: you feel it, therefore it must be true.
(8) 'Should' statements: musts and oughts. You feel as if you have to whip yourself before you can do anything. Mmmmm. Musterbation.
(9) Labelling and mislabelling: 'I am a loser'; 'He is a louse.'
(10) Personalisation: you see yourself as the cause of some negative personal event for which you were not responsible.

So I'm depressed. Still. Oh, and I still loathe the word 'catastrophising'.

Then the King George V Fund for Actors sends me a cheque. I weep my thanks unashamedly down the phone to the actors Julian Glover and Geraldine McEwan who've been the motors behind it, but I am ashamed that I have no idea why King George V (bless him) should have been so partial to actors. I'm just soggily grateful that he was—as well as those who came after him with their bequests and legacies. I trek through clothes shops spending real and imaginary fortunes to clothe my ever-expanding backside. I give myself challenges of how polite I can be in shops when I am dropping with exhaustion because, yes, I have overdone it. The answer is still— polite? 'Not very.'

My ancient friend of the periwinkle-blue eyes, darling Floy, says someone remarked about me in the village shop. She has told me this story before but I don't let on. 'And I said, "Well, you know, she has been *very ill.*" But I think you're getting better, darling, because you know, you're not so . . . not so . . . oh, what's the right word? You'll kill me if I get it wrong. You're not so *abrasive.*'

Dear Doc Lewith asks me to give a speech at the Royal College of Physicians annual conference on 'Allopathic and homeopathic medicine from the patients' point of view.' I have enough ammunition: eyes, womb, back, shoulder, hip and brain. I speak in front of two hundred medics, and abrasive is exactly what I am.

A month or so later though I find I have written 'I feel as if I've turned another corner.' These corners aren't easily definable in the healing process: they're an almost imperceptible change of gear. Something shifts internally. I am slower. I feel when I need to stop. I don't rush if I can help it. It's as if another section of my brain, perhaps, has relaxed, has stopped its swollen chafing against my skull. I certainly don't scratch my scalp as fiendishly as I once did. My head still whines and whizzes, though, especially if I turn quickly. Occasionally a sharp sliver of pain makes me squawk. It catches me involuntarily. I react to it out loud, wherever I am. It has a way of clearing a path in front of me in crowds. Useful.

I'm not quite so rattled on the tube, these days—or, at least, I can measure my degree of rattledness as equal to the degree of exhaustion quite clearly now. I have carried the feel-good book around with me for weeks, like the Holy Grail, mostly with its covers bent back. Sometimes I hide it inside the *Guardian*, although I can't take much of the pain in the news of the external world. I am religiously doing all the exercises in the book. Learning how to analyse a situation that caused me grief and seeing which of these ten points was in action. Sometimes I score as high as six. It is a revelation to me. I read that no one seems to know whether depression is caused by too little or too much serotonin. I am absorbed by the side-effects of anti-depressants (at least the SSRIs not the MAOIs): dry mouth and throat, headache, tiredness, insomnia, upset stomach, constipation, blurred vision, lightheadedness, confusion, anxiety, dizziness. I had all these before I started taking the tablets. I have most of them still. I thought that was what they were supposed to *cure*.

At least the book stops me glaring at people on trains.

Coincidentally, the GP from Warwickshire rings about the prescription for the anti-depressants soon coming to an end, and asks if I'm still seeing my 'psychiatric nurse'. I am affronted by the misnomer from somebody in the business, and fiercely reject the slur on my mental health.

'*The neuro-psychologist?*' I say, rather pointedly. 'Yes, and she and the hospital advise that I keep on taking the anti-depressants, thank you.' I put the phone down with a smash.

Several days later I buy a fridge magnet for the Godsend that says, 'One in three people are unbalanced. Think of two friends. If they seem OK, you're the one.' He sticks it on my fridge.

The Godsend comes to a neuro-psychology session with me. I am overjoyed. This feels right. I'm always seeing husbands or wives, partners of people who've been felled by a stroke, or some brain bomb, lending an arm or pushing a wheelchair, or encouraging first shaky steps on a walking-frame around the hospital's reception area. He's somewhat hesitant because I was stupid enough to blurt out that Dr Baehr had been rather concerned about a new relationship while I am still, as she would put it, 'in recovery'. When I go to the support group at the hospital I see why. Two of the patients, both 'in recovery', have discovered each other. There is something quite disarming about their apparent delight in each other. It is also rather naive and worryingly euphoric.

The Godsend wants to know from Dr Baehr what he's doing wrong. There is no question of wrong, as far as I'm concerned. This man has heard me scream and sob, and HBO people, although luckily he seems to be exempt himself. He has witnessed voluble panic-attacks and once he actually had to stop me banging my head against the wall when I was in despair at the slowness and confusion of my new brain. I would lick the mud off his shoes for the love and care he shows me, but his shoes are always polished shining bright.

Dr Baehr asks him what he means by wrong.

'Well, for example, what do I do when she starts having blanks—when she's trying to find words—or when she slurs and stutters them out? It's wrong to help her out with the words she's searching for, isn't it?'

I wait for her reply with interest. It's only since we've been close that there is a day-to-day monitoring of my behaviour.

'If she's stuttering and blanking out, she's gone too far. Neither of you should have let her get to that stage of exhaustion.'

I say to the Godsend as we are about to leave something I have been told, but never said, 'Do *you* know just how *lucky* I am? If this had happened to me in England there is no doubt I would be dead.'

We go to a crowded wedding near Pisa. I can't not go. It's my son's very first girlfriend of whom I am very fond; I'd hoped she would be my daughter-in-law. She has asked me to recite a John Donne poem for her. The Godsend and I spend two happy days, he exploring the botany at the edge of the bay while I walk up and down the beach topping up my tan and learning my lines, or 'overlearning' as Dr Baehr would describe it. Then it's easier to 'pull-up'. The wedding itself, though magnificent, is too much of everything for my bewildered travel-strained brain. "Too many people, too much music, too many bright lights, too much talk. We survive it, just. I am querulous, picky and difficult, unbalanced after the flight and disturbed by so much stimulus. I retreat to a seat in the shadow of the veranda. I feel old. The other me wants to get up and dance and whirl and whoop and utterly let go.

We have a delightful day to ourselves on our way back to England. We arrive in Pisa just as the Tower has been reopened after engineering works to strengthen it. We don't go up it. We don't need to. Just sitting on the grass, admiring it from many angles, makes my sense of balance go quite doo-lally. We dawdle home that night along the banks of the Arno, with the other stragglers who are enjoying the velvet blackness of the midsummer sky. In the middle of a bridge further along, a middle-aged choir, dressed in silver spangles, sing all the middle-of-the-road tacky numbers from the seventies in very Italianised English. We join in and sing, shameless that we know the words: 'You, you make me feel brand new, /Oh, God bless you-oo-oo . . .'

We giggle and fart about like sixteen-year-olds. Well, I am, of course.

In England, only days later, I read in the newspaper, 'Researchers from Pisa have categorised romantic palpitations as chemically akin to compulsive-obsessive disorder. Both spring from very low levels of the neuro-transmitter serotonin.' Oh, well. Perhaps I should double up on the pills.

I have been advised—no, warned—by Dr Baehr that on the few occasions that I work with other actors, and not on my own in a recital, to remember that I've 'come to do a job. It's not about how smart you are, or how stupid they are.' I seem to see through people still. Their motives seem transparent. It's as if, having lost my top layer of skin, I see beyond and beneath it in others too. It's very disconcerting. I certainly see through myself.

In one session I ask her, 'Do you think brain damage makes people psychic?'

There is an uncommonly long pause before she answers, very emphatically, 'No.' I sense it's not just an answer: it is loaded with warning.

When I ask that question again, in the second support group I go to at the NHS

355

hospital, again thanks to BASIC, almost a year after my initial visit, the husband of one of the original patients I met laughs in response to my query and says, 'Psychic? You should take more water with it.'

Indeed, Dr Baehr has said I should dilute wine with water. My stepfather, who taught me the pleasures of good wine, would turn in his Parisian grave. Tiredness plus two glasses of wine, and I lose all my short-term memory, my tact, and social niceties.

There are several faces I recognise at this meeting, including the nurse who was in charge of the group last time. She no longer works at the hospital but still comes to help the group. She recognises me as the woman who got up and left last time I was there because I couldn't stand the noise. I tell her quietly outside in a corridor that I am trying to write a book about brain haemorrhage. She is immediately defensive and protective of the people in the group. 'No, no, absolutely not. These people are here in trust.'

'But I'm not doing anything disloyal. I'm hoping this book will help.'

'No, you mustn't. They're here incognito.'

'I shan't use any names.'

'No, you can't.'

'But I'm a brain patient *too*. I *know* what it's like. I won't betray them.' I think, This is absurd. *I'm* one of *them*. I am already trembling with anger and frustration. I can't

356

believe she doesn't see she's making me worse. We have locked horns. Neither of us is going to give in.

I go into the room. There are six or seven people. The nurse starts the meeting by introducing an administrator who wants the group's input into the design of a new neurological ward that's planned for this hospital. I'm so wound up by the set-to in the corridor that I charge in: 'The NHS needs more doctors and nurses—more *people* trained —not buildings.'

They all look surprised at my outburst. I can see that they were initially flattered to be asked. I see that request for the sop it is. I am on the roller-coaster and I can't get off. 'How many of you have done a neuro-psychology test?' I ask.

No one.

'How many of you saw a neuro-psychologist?'

None.

'Have you?' someone says.

'Yes. I . . . er . . . I pay for it.'

Which is true, in a sort of way. But this answer alienates me even more than my manner of speaking. I don't have the guts to say I have private sickness cover. My foster-mother, a staunch Labour voter all her life, looms large of a sudden.

'How many neuro-psychologists *are* there in this hospital?' It was my understanding that this was one of the biggest of all neurological hospitals in London.

The administrator says, 'One.'

It is shocking. We are all silent.

'And he's at full stretch most days from seven thirty in the morning to eight o'clock at night.'

'Why did none of you get to see him?'

'Because we haven't got any deficits,' seems to be the consensus. I am shocked. 'What— you mean he only sees people who can't walk or can't talk?'

'Yes.'

A strong-looking chap, who'd described himself as a builder when we'd all had to introduce ourselves, says, 'I was tipped out of here after just five days. Five days.' He shakes his head sadly. 'I thought I was going mad.'

All of us nod. We murmur in recognition. We know.

Later, in the car as he gives me a lift home, he says, 'It was terrible. I just used to sit and cry.' It is more poignant because he is stockily built, a burly chap who wouldn't look out of place as a nightclub bouncer. 'I was frightened. I was frightened to go out. Frightened to go to the shops. Frightened even to cross the bloody road.' His son, who lives with him, has bought him a puppy. 'I'm all right now because I got my lovely dog. I just sit at home and cuddle my dog. But I was frightened. Frightened of everything.'

CHAPTER TWENTY-FOUR

More Circles

I do manage to get on a stage. A stage I helped
for fifteen years to build. It never fails to thrill
me when I walk into its yard. In the summer I
present the Globe award to John Barton,
a much-loved, much-revered teacher of
Shakespeare. He is frail and fragile from a
recent bug and I delight in running about
making sure he has enough to eat and drink. It
is still a new experience for me to be looking
after someone else and I relish it to the full.
But my own illness has taught me that there
are boundaries to helping. In the wings,
though he is calm—he has decided not to
make a speech—I am at war within myself, a
mixture of alarm and envy: alarm at having to
speak in front of over a thousand people; envy
as we are waiting with the actors who are
beginners in *Lear* and who will start playing
the play as soon as my speech is over. I
whisper, 'I want to look after you enough so
that you feel safe and supported, but I don't
want to invade your privacy or your dignity.'

'Quite so,' he says.

Well, I know well.

As I help him into the taxi afterwards,
making the driver promise not to let him leave

the award on the back seat, he says, 'It was great to see you take the stage. You paced about it like a lion. You couldn't have done that a year ago.'

I miss my job. I miss the theatre. I have a yearning for it, like the yearning one has for an absent lover. I have had to turn down many theatre jobs, simply because I cannot manage the demands of eight performances a week, with two on a mid-week day and two on a Saturday. My agent comforts me by pointing out that at least the work is still coming my way. And I take one more step forward, work-wise.

I do a solo performance of poetry. A full-length performance all on my own with an interval in the middle. I remember how it felt a year ago to be standing in the same room at the Shakespeare Centre in Stratford. Norman has died from a brain haemorrhage since I stood here last. A cruel piece of synchronicity. My dear Floy has died too. I have the periwinkle-blue scarf back. It smells of her special perfume. I dedicate poems to them both.

This time my head is connected to my body, and I feel connected through my feet to the stage. I have worked and worked on the poems, many of which I almost know by head and by heart. There are many friends in the audience who are aware of how significant this evening is for me and my recovery. Ray and Nev and Sue and Adrian have come all the way from Bristol. And my new family, Philip and Harriet and Auntie Margaret. As I walk out on to the stage the adrenaline hits me. I remember Dr Baehr asking, when I was grieving over the loss of the Callas role, why didn't I do just a couple of speeches from it in my sitting room at home? This is why, Dr Baehr: three hundred or so people out for the evening, waiting, watching, wanting to enjoy themselves. All the best work comes from actors being a mouthpiece for the writer's words and thoughts. It has nothing to do with showing off, which is all ego. It has everything to do with no ego at all, by being a vessel through which the writer speaks. An instrument. A link between writer and listener. I love every single moment of it. I hear some of the poems I know well in a way I've never heard them before. I'm not playing them. They are playing me. I feel fully alive in a way I haven't felt for a long, long time.

It seems a small price to pay, the inevitable few days of feeling dead that follow it. Death seems all around. No Floy to pop in to see, with a dish of her favourite egg custard, that is hard. There is a Floy-shaped gap in the village. I grieve. I also have pangs about Norman not surviving what I did. That's a hard one too.

Coincidentally the next chapter in the feel-good book is the hardest: 'Your Work Is Not Your Worth.' Yes, well. We know about the Protestant work ethic. We know about the way the marketplace quantifies people by what they do, not who they are. But what about us lucky few who love our work? I skip through this chapter, not really taking much notice. I put away the poetry file with some sadness. My next recital isn't till Christmas. Then it will be almost two years AC.

The length of time doesn't shock me any more. My grasp on time is different now. Actually I don't think I have a grasp at all.

Dr Baehr is encouraging about my charts: they show that I am handling a lot more stress—my own, not other people's—a lot of travelling to and fro, from London mostly, to teach the odd class at the Actors' Centre or to record a radio play. I'm not feeling so ill, just empty. But I seem to have stuck at three half-mornings of work a week, or two consecutive days. Anything more than that and I'm in trouble. The only difference between now and a year ago is that I'm unwilling to push myself harder. I want to stay within what Dr Baehr describes as the comfort zone. My sleep is still erratic and sporadic. I get up now and read or watch the dawn streak the sky with light. I spend ages at the window, just looking. Something I haven't done since I was a child.

I have stopped being quite so obsessed by children. I notice that I'm not as aware of them as I was. Not so in tune with what every facial gesture is meant to convey. Perhaps my brain is growing up at last.

I'm still rubbing friends up the wrong way. I meet Darleney after I've been teaching at the Globe. A three-hour class with undergraduates is demanding and consequently draining. My energy level is utterly depleted and Darleney, as it happens, is stressed, confused and depressed. Her discomfort bleeds into me as if I were a sheet of blotting paper. I have no defences against it.

I try to help her by forcing my mind to apply itself to her various problems, which of course I cannot do so I end up being scratchy with her and irritated by her. The rawness in the chest comes back and the pain between the shoulder-blades makes itself felt anew.

'Why should you have to cope with her stress?' asks Dr Baehr, later. 'You are still learning to manage your own.'

'Well, because she was kind enough to help *me*.'

'Yes, but pushing your brain like that when you're tired—it's like trying to walk on a broken leg.'

I wince. That's a sharp image.

'You are still—'

'I'm still convalescent. I know.'

'You are still *in recovery*.' This has become a

363

running gag between us now. 'You are still in recovery. Don't forget that.'

'But I do. Other people do, too. It's harder now that I'm almost well. People don't ask how I am any more. They're bored with it. I'm bored with it.' And for the millionth time, I cry.

Dr Baehr suggests discussing the dose of anti-depressant with my GP as I still exhibit signs of major depression. I despair. I feel a total failure. My son is kind and supportive about it. 'It is, after all, an illness, Ma. You're being treated for an illness. Look at it that way.'

I hear an old script: 'But my mother was a depressive. And my mother was a failure. A failure as my mother and a failure as a person.'

He knows the repartee, even if I leave this step out: 'You are not your mother.'

I wish I'd said, 'No, my dear son, and neither are you mine.' But his tenderness towards me is so new, and of such value, I daren't risk it. Anyway, if there's any mothering going I'm still up for it. Or fathering.

The Godsend promises to monitor my behaviour. To see if there is any change at all in me with the double dose of pills.

I ring Darleney, who's now working, apologise and explain that it is part of my illness, not being able to handle other people's stress.

'Well, I'm still in the same situation as I was then,' she says. The implication being that I'm handling it all right now.

'No, you're not,' I counter. 'You've just told me you've got work.' Actor's shorthand for 'So everything is now all right.'

It is several months and two cards from me before I hear from her again. The ripple effect still weaves its magic spell, then.

None of my friends ask me any more if I have work. That in itself speaks volumes. I have no work. So I am not all right.

Occasionally, especially now I'm writing—which demands great concentration and painful emotional recall—I can still end up on the floor, wrung out and wretched. Dr Baehr's damage control comes into play when I encounter the ground:

—Don't speak to anyone on the phone—unplug it.

—Watch how much wine I drink. Tiredness and alcohol are a potent mixture. Not only do I lose track of what I'm doing, I lose track of what I'm saying too, and can come out with some real stinkers.

—Don't go shopping.

—Don't socialise.

—Don't deal with any big issues.

Stay in my burrow.

The Godsend catches me singing in the kitchen as I'm cooking, and gives me a knowing look. I'm always happy when I'm cooking and now I cook almost every day. It's a welcome break from the rigours of writing, doing something practical with my hands. It never feels like work. In a kitchen I feel close to the French grandmother I never knew. He holds my gaze.

'Why are you looking at me like that? Oh, is it because—'

'Yes. You're better.'

'Oh, no.'

' 'Fraid so. Keep taking the tablets.'

I throw the wet dishcloth at him. It hits the mark.

A moment of crisis. My third laptop crash in three weeks. I have already lost two thousand words. Twice before I have jumped on a train to London and taken it back to the repair shop. Impulsive, *moi*? Even with the expert's know-how the words stay resolutely lost. 'User error' is their diagnosis. The residue of tiredness builds. I ring Dr Baehr at the hospital. I need her cool head and calm voice.

'Can I speak to Dr Baehr, please?'

'She's not here.'

'Oh . . . well, can I speak to her secretary?'

'She's not here.'

That's odd. It is, after all, three o'clock in the afternoon on a weekday.

'Well, can I speak to anyone in the neuro-psychology department?'

'It's not here.'

My grasp on reality begins to wobble. 'Hang on. I've been coming for treatment there for nearly a year. I'm not mad.' Am I? No.

With renewed conviction I continue, 'Damn it all, I even opened the new department there in August.' Didn't I? I said the Guillaume Apollinaire poem for Dr Baehr at the end of the speech:

> Come to the edge
> No, we are frightened
> Come to the edge
> We will fall
> Come to the edge
> They came
> And she pushed them
> And they flew.

I say, as if to convince myself, 'There's a plaque on the wall with my name on it.'

'Well, the department's not here. I mean all the equipment's here. But the department's not here any more.'

'What?' I shout.

'This is an old people's home. An old people's home. It always was.'

I call Dr Baehr on her mobile.

Dr Baehr feels that I am making great strides and suggests a new plan of campaign

367

for me now is to get out and about in my working world again. I go to an awards ceremony at the National Theatre. It's a small guest list of actors who all know each other, a comfortable experience and a great lunch. I'm rather shaky as I dress up—avoiding the clothes I no longer fit into. Stress limitation. I put on my war-paint. I know there will be many friends there whom I haven't seen for nearly two years, BC and AC.

I bump into one in the loo, as I repair the damage from the treat of the taxi journey. We have been *so* worried about you,' she says. I have had one phone call and a postcard from her in two years. How worried can you get? I say nothing. That's progress.

In a lull in the proceedings an old girlfriend of my ex-husband comes over to the table I am on. I haven't seen her since the day she handed my then nine-year-old son over to me on the doorstep of my marital home, after a weekend he had spent with her and his father, with advice about what I must do for his cold. Twenty years ago. She sits down in the empty seat beside me and, with big eyes, says, 'How *are* you?'

I take a deep breath mentally, and quietly reply, 'Go away.'

'What have I ever done to you?' she asks, taken aback.

'Go away,' I say again. Quiet but firm.

She goes, muttering something about

a shame.

I think it a triumph.

I can't wait to relate it to Dr Baehr.

Cognitive therapy—yes.

Ends are being tied off. Circles are being completed.

I have a chance to be reaquainted with my beloved Katharine of Aragon, albeit briefly. Greg Doran is filming four TV programmes of RSC actors doing bits of Shakespeare. I haven't worn a theatre costume for two and a half years. A four-inch gusset has to be put into one of Katharine's dresses so that the lacing at the back will meet. It was in Washington DC at the Kennedy Center in 1998 that I said goodbye to her.

For days I go over and over and over the lines. I can't afford to dry—there will be a lot of actors hanging around whom I haven't seen since before . . .

I will always remember the moment that Dr Vinikoff told me that my chances of pulling through the operation were slight. My clear and uncluttered reaction was, I've been an actor. I've been to places that most people never get to see, I've met some extraordinary people. Indeed.

I play Katharine in the Great Hall at Hampton Court, in the kind of clothes she would have worn when she herself was in that room. It is eerie. Excitingly so. My new, larger body copes with the weight of the velour, velvet and dévoré with fur sleeves that reach to the floor better than my old frail, stress-ridden one did. The Godsend hears the applause. I feel strong as a lion.

CHAPTER TWENTY-FIVE

The End of the Beginning

Two and a half years on from 11 January 2000, life is not as vivid as it was. The whole experience, I feel, is now 'over there'. But then again the pain of it is not so acute either. My brain feels as if at last it is back inside my head. The headaches aren't too bad now. That's partly due to the one 25-mg night-time amitriptyline that I now take—an old-fashioned anti-depressant, well tried and tested, that apparently has a calming effect on pain.

The recent MRI scans were OK, but this time I cried on coming out of the tunnel of pneumatic drills. I do pee less now, so maybe my stepfather was right.

Mr Kitchen's statistics were right about the second aneurysm not going: 20 per cent of half a per cent. I don't mind being one of that herd. I have finally left the Warwickshire GP. No letter was sent. Sadly my London GP has retired so I was forced into finding a replacement here in the country. I have. He is kind, attentive and understanding, and he's NHS. I *am* lucky.

Through the Godsend I have experienced a new state: contentment. From time to time we both forget that my still-new brain can get very tired. Cerebral irritation. There are days when I could irrit for England.

My collection of furry animals has grown unashamedly. The child lives on quite comfortably inside me now, no longer broken off. But on bad days the Shadow rules and it is not OK.

I still don't know whether I'll ever be able to manage eight shows a week again. It's a bit like a plangent refrain that I hear when I'm low. But it is getting fainter all the time.

Time, as I have heard non-stop for the last two and a half years, will tell. Never say never.

Ironically the pension company have axed 25 per cent of my monthly income because of the little bit of part-time work that I have been doing. But so far, in the last six months, it's been one of the starkest times I've ever had professionally, though I had this book to blunt the sting of unemployment. When I started this I couldn't sit at it for more than twenty minutes without my head reeling. Now I can write off and on for most of the working day, as long as I take Dr Baehr's recommended breaks every twenty minutes or so. I still have wasp-like head zaps and whines, but I read them as warning signs of imminent HBO state and exhaustion collapse imminent. STOP NOW. I have learned to take care of myself—with more than a little help from my friends. I listen to my body. ME exists: official. So, it's all right to be wretched. I couldn't resist sending the newspaper articles that gave it credence to the Prof who wouldn't admit it exists—I didn't hear from her. I wasn't surprised.

I have lost four film jobs in a row. One after the other. My confidence is smashed. I have decided since October 2002 not to put myself up for any film or TV work at all.

Perhaps work-wise the word has got round that I am, have been, was ill? The business is a fickle swine.

The background worry of having my pension axed has shot my blood pressure up into the danger zone. What a joke. I survived death because I have—or, at least, I used to have—low blood pressure. I walk half an hour a day. I don't smoke. I don't drink as much red wine, and still we can't get the damn hypertension out of the danger zone. I know a lot about living with fear. But it causes me stress. I don't like being stressed any more. My new brain can't manage it. What was all the pain for, if I haven't learned from it?

As a test, to see what I am capable of now, with Dr Baehr's input, I have just completed three half-days of teaching for two weeks, and a whole half-week of teaching at Balliol plus two poetry recitals, one in Norfolk and a five-hour drive either end. I was utterly depleted by it. This tested Nerves of Steel to his utmost.

Me too.

I checked in with Dr Baehr, as she wanted to review me following this increase in work. The outcome was that a full return to work may be unrealistic.

I didn't cry.

My son and I are as close as we ever were, with a difference. We have both lived through this very real upheaval that threatened our relationship and have come out the other side with another, deeper dimension of understanding between us.

I can't say I am more patient, but I can say I know when I am impatient. And why. I'm lucky. I am about as lucky as anyone can get.

We called in at Peterborough Cathedral on our way back from the recital in Norfolk. I said thank you to Catalina one more time, and left a flower. Things do seem to have come full circle.

I asked for strength to endure at the Quaker retreat. It seems, blessedly, that it was granted me.

My hour of silence each Sunday is essential, and my quiet times during the week a solace and a sanctuary. I have Time now.

The priest said that one day I would look

back on all this as a blessing.

The hardest thing of all which made my sense of injustice boil and rage, was being judged on behaviour for which I was not responsible, over which I had no control.

I have grieved a lot in these last three years. Not least of all for the mother I never had, the foster-mother I miss still, and the father I never knew.

There is a moment at the end of the play about Callas where, as she finishes teaching her masterclass, she walks round the stage and takes one last lingering look into the auditorium, knowing it will be the last time she ever stands on stage. I often think back to that. Each time I did it. How real it seemed.

Lucky, grateful, slower, fatter and wiser. I don't regret a day of it. I mean, I have never wished it hadn't happened. When I have crises—and I still do—I remember Dr Baehr's words—you don't go back to the beginning, you just get off the path for a while. It has given me a better life. I don't have as much of lots of the things I had before, but I have more of what I never had. As they say in the theatre, less is more. What a paradox.

Glossary

BASIC   Brain and Spinal Injuries Charity
CAT   Computerised Axial Tomography
ECT   Electro-convulsive therapy
EEG   Electro-encephalogram
MAOI   Monoamine Oxidase Inhibitor
MRI   Magnetic Resonance Imaging
SAH   Subarachnoid haemorrhage
SSRI   Selective Serotonin Re-uptake
          Inhibitors

Helpful Addresses

BASIC

Brain and Spinal Injuries Charity
The Neurocare Centre
554 Eccles New Road
Salford
Manchester M5 1AL
email: basic-charity@compuserve.com

Headway—The Brain Injury Association
4 King Edward Street
Nottingham HGI IEW
Tel: 0115 924 0800
email: enquiries@headway.org.uk
www.headway.org.uk

British Brain And Spine Foundaiton
7 Winchester House
Kennington Park
Cranmer Road
London SW9 6EJ
Tel: 0207 793 5909
Helpline: 0808 808 1000
email: helpline@bbsf.org.uk
www.tna-uk.org.uk

Rehabilitation Network
1 Lindsay House
5-9 Gloucester Road
London SW7 4PP
Tel: 0207 467 8575
email:rnetuk@aol.com
www.rehabnetwork.info